BUS

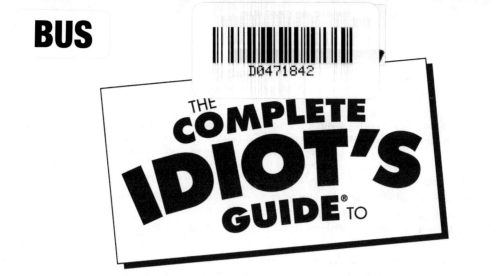

THE
COMPLETE IDIOT'S GUIDE® TO

Sports Nutrition

by Dawn Weatherwax, ATC/L, RD, CSCS and Sonia Weiss

ALPHA

A member of Penguin Group (USA) Inc.

International Standard Book Number: 1-59257-102-6
Library of Congress Catalog Card Number: 2003108341

05   04   03   8   7   6   5   4   3   2   1

Interpretation of the printing code: The rightmost number of the first series of numbers is the year of the book's printing; the rightmost number of the second series of numbers is the number of the book's printing. For example, a printing code of 03-1 shows that the first printing occurred in 2003.

Printed in the United States of America

Note: This publication contains the opinions and ideas of its authors. It is intended to provide helpful and informative material on the subject matter covered. It is sold with the understanding that the authors and publisher are not engaged in rendering professional services in the book. If the reader requires personal assistance or advice, a competent professional should be consulted.

The authors and publisher specifically disclaim any responsibility for any liability, loss, or risk, personal or otherwise, which is incurred as a consequence, directly or indirectly, of the use and application of any of the contents of this book.

Publisher: *Marie Butler-Knight*
Product Manager: *Phil Kitchel*
Senior Managing Editor: *Jennifer Chisholm*
Senior Acquisitions Editor: *Mike Sanders*
Senior Development Editor: *Michael Thomas*
Production Editor: *Billy Fields*
Copy Editor: *Jan Zoya*
Illustrator: *Chris Eliopoulos*
Cover/Book Designer: *Trina Wurst*
Indexer: *Heather McNeill*
Layout/Proofreading: *John Etchison, Rebecca Harmon*

Contents at a Glance

Contents

Foreword

In 25 years as a strength and conditioning professional I have trained thousands of athletes. Despite earnest efforts and disciplined adherence to well-designed programs, many athletes fail to improve the way they should. Factors such as genetics, illness, and poor lifestyle decisions are sometimes to blame; but the most common reason for their frustration is their nutritional status.

We have all heard of athletes who eat horrible diets yet perform at very high levels. These are exceptions to the norm that often serve as justification to athletes who choose to eat a less-than-ideal diet. The fact is, the vast majority of athletes can greatly improve their health and physical capacity by changing at least some of the ways and some of the things they eat.

Building a great body is similar to building a house. In both cases basic components are assembled in varying quantities and combinations following a predetermined pattern. Can you imagine trying to build a house without the right number of bricks or the right kind of electrical wire? What if you had plenty of paint, but it was all pink? Or you wanted a three-car garage, but you had only two garage doors?

Working out, practicing, and competing stress the body in ways that cause it to try to adapt. The human body, unlike other machines that wear out, can actually get better as you use it. Exercise signals the body to follow its genetic blueprint to produce new and better molecules and cells more suited to performing at a higher level. This growth and development occurs only when the materials needed to support it are present in the appropriate quantities. In addition to building materials, large amounts of energy are required to fuel the high levels of exertion typical of athletes and to sustain the growth and repair process that is the heart of physical improvement.

If the contractor building a house runs short on materials, he or she can simply visit the local hardware store and pick up the appropriate supplies. That is not the case for the human body. If it is lacking an essential nutrient, something does not happen—or at least, it does not happen well. The body's stores of key compounds, vitamins, minerals, and water are limited to what is taken in by the athlete. A poor diet can easily be as limiting to an athlete's success as a bad training program or a lack of adherence to their coach's and/or trainer's instructions.

If you want to improve your athletic ability, or that of your child or someone else you are working with, this should be the next book you read. There is a wealth of in-depth information on these pages, but there are also plenty of simple tips to make improving your diet easy. Most people can greatly improve their nutritional status by changing as few as three to five things about the way they eat. The trick is determining the areas that need to be addressed. This book not only identifies the essential needs of the athlete, it does so in a manner that is convincing and understandable. Following even the most basic principles contained in this book should improve any athlete's performance and greatly enhance their chances of good health.

—Joe Owens, MS, CSCS*D
Director of Athletic Performance Enhancement
University of Dayton, Dayton, Ohio

Introduction

Eat right, and get enough rest and exercise. This has been the basic prescription for good health since antiquity. The ancient Greeks and Romans understood that all three principles could both cause ill health and cure it, and their words ring as true today as they did centuries ago. When we balance these elements in our life, we simply feel better, look better, and perform better. Who could ask for anything more?

This balance is what sports nutrition is all about. It takes nutrition to the next level by combining all three principles to help everyone bring out the best in him- or herself—the "athlete within." Because sports nutrition takes into account individual needs, goals, and objectives, it truly works for everyone—world-class athletes, weekend warriors, senior Olympians, Little Leaguers—you name it.

So don't let the title of this book put you off for even a second. If you move your body and you eat—and who doesn't?—you can use the principles of sports nutrition to optimize your nutrition, and, in turn, optimize your workouts, practices, events, classes, and even your everyday activities. You'll make the time you spend being active the very best it can be. In the pages that follow, you'll be well on your way to putting together your own plan for optimal fitness and wellness.

In **Part 1, "The Training Table,"** you'll learn about the basics of sports nutrition and how it differs from regular nutrition. We'll also talk about how your body uses the nutrients you put into it and discuss the habits that can make good nutrition a part of your life.

Part 2, "Ready! Set! Eat Well!" discusses the nuts and bolts of basic nutrition. In this part, you'll learn about macronutrients and micronutrients—the building blocks of the food you eat—and why eating them in the right proportions can have such a big impact on what you do both on and off the athletic field.

Part 3, "Hitting the Food Trail," gives you the specifics for crafting a sports-nutrition program. In this part, you'll learn how to stock your shelves right, how to buy vitamins and supplements, how to eat on the go, and how to eat for optimal performance, both before and after games, practices, and workouts.

In **Part 4, "Athletes In All Shapes and Sizes,"** we discuss the specific nutritional needs of various types of athletes, including men, women, children, vegetarians, and seniors.

Part 5, "Nutrition for Special Needs," shows you how to put your sports-nutrition knowledge to work in special situations such as losing weight, gaining muscle, and getting back on your feet after illness or injury.

Finally, at the end of the book you'll find two helpful appendixes that contain a list of the terms used in this book, and further resources.

Extras

To help you get the most out of *The Complete Idiot's Guide to Sports Nutrition*, you'll find more information on various aspects of sports nutrition in the following information boxes:

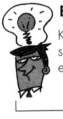

Eat It Up!

Key information, tips, and suggestions on eating and exercise.

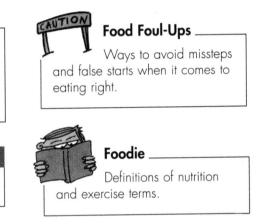

Food Foul-Ups

Ways to avoid missteps and false starts when it comes to eating right.

Dawn Says

Advice straight from the expert.

Foodie

Definitions of nutrition and exercise terms.

Acknowledgments

From Dawn:

First I want to thank the Almighty for bringing me this opportunity.

Next, I'm grateful to my parents for always supporting me in my endeavors throughout adolescence until now. I have sure tested their patience and love at times.

A special thanks to my agent, Jessica Faust, for answering numerous questions and putting up with my naïve nature.

I want to acknowledge people who have had a pivotal impact on my life: Coach Limbach, Kathy English, Karen Moses, Dr. Melinda Manore, Melvin Douglas, and Ellen Schuman.

I am also grateful for Tremayne Miller, Stephanie Tevis, and Anthony Willert, who helped gather information for the book, and to Rita Heikenfeld for providing so many great recipes.

I want to say thanks to all my long-lasting friends who have supported me through all the years—Stacie Pennington, Dori Hunt, Cassie Samuelson, Dana Crumbly, Debbie Reyher, and Kent Pilakowski.

A special note to my sister Clairinda who puts up with my endless chatter on a regular basis, and a sisterly love/friendship I never imagined we would have. To my brother Brian who is always in my corner. And lastly to my love, DJ, who put up with my absence and lack of companionship on top of my already hectic schedule.

I am on my hands and knees with praise to Sonia Weiss, my co-author. She made the process of writing a book as painless as it can possibly be. Her ability to take my information and make it fun and readable is amazing. She is wonderful to work with.

Finally, endless thanks to Rita Heikenfeld, who can take regular recipes, change them to be fit for sports performance, and make them taste great. Every athlete who has used her recipes, young and old, has raved about them and they always want more.

From Sonia:

A big thanks to Jessica Faust and Jacky Sach at Bookends, Inc., for pairing me with such a great co-author. Not only was she a delight to work with, this lady knows what she's talking about! Also many thanks to the editorial and production team at Alpha Books, including Mike Sanders, Mike Thomas, Billy Fields, and Jan Zoya, for their help in getting all the pieces in the right places. Thanks also go to Roy White at the General Merchandise Distributors Council for his assistance on information pertaining to supermarket shopping and shopping trends.

Trademarks

All terms mentioned in this book that are known to be or are suspected of being trademarks or service marks have been appropriately capitalized. Alpha Books and Penguin Group (USA) Inc. cannot attest to the accuracy of this information. Use of a term in this book should not be regarded as affecting the validity of any trademark or service mark.

Part 1

The Training Table

Sports nutrition takes good nutrition and rachets it up a step. It focuses on using the food you eat to fuel your performance, regardless of what you do. If you are a competitive runner trying to improve your stamina and times, sports nutrition will help you attain your goals. Proper nutrient intake can increase your performance from 5 to 15 percent. You can't beat an edge like this! If you enjoy working out because of how it makes you look and feel, knowing what and when to eat can make the time you spend exercising pay off even better.

In this part, you'll learn about the basics of sports nutrition and how it differs from regular nutrition. We'll also talk about how your body uses the nutrients you put into it and discuss the habits that can make good nutrition a part of your life.

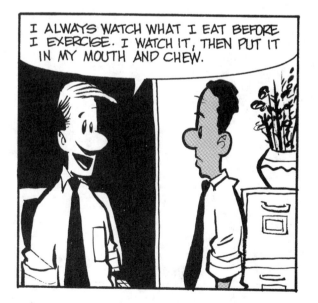

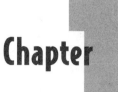

The Starting Line

In This Chapter

- ◆ Eating to live
- ◆ Early nutritional discoveries
- ◆ Nutrition as science
- ◆ The evolution of sports nutrition

Everyone knows that you have to eat to live, right? With maybe a few exceptions—there are reports of yogis and other highly austere religious types who exist on nothing but air—taking in food is an essential of life. Most people have to chomp down on something on a fairly regular basis to keep functioning. As long as we live, we need to eat.

But there is a difference between shoveling in calories and eating wisely. As an athlete, you probably already know this. What you may not know, however, is why eating right can make such a big difference in your performance.

Beginning with the Basics

We're going to start our exploration of sports nutrition with a few assumptions. We're going to assume that you are not an air-eating yogi and that you get your fuel from food.

Since you have picked up this book, we are also going to assume that the subject of sports nutrition intrigues you for some reason. Maybe you're a pretty fair amateur athlete who wants to know more about how nutrition can improve your performance. Maybe you're the parent of a young athlete and you want to safeguard your child from sports-related injuries through good nutritional practices. Or maybe you're a formerly active person who wants to get back into the action and you know that eating well can help you do it. But, with all the conflicting information out there about what a good diet is all about, you're not sure what eating well even means anymore.

Regardless of which category you fit into, and, of course, there are many more that we haven't even mentioned here, understanding the basics of good nutrition is definitely a good investment in your overall health. And understanding the basics of sports nutrition is a good investment in your athletic performance.

Nutrition vs. Sports Nutrition

Nutrition is a hot topic these days. It seems like there is a new report issued almost every day on some aspect of food and how it affects the body—either positively or negatively. Because we hear so much about nutrition, it might come as a surprise to learn that the formal science of nutrition—and sports nutrition, for that matter—are relatively new. In fact, the term nutrition did not even come into popular use until the late 1800s. The term sports nutrition came along much later—not until the middle of the twentieth century.

Foodie

Nutrition is defined as a science that deals with foods and their effect on health. Add sports to the equation, and you have a science that deals with foods and how they affect the health—and, subsequently, the performance—of athletes. Sports nutrition combines knowledge from the separate but related fields of nutrition and exercise.

Both sciences are based on centuries of inquiry and research in the areas of medicine, anatomy, biology, chemistry, physics, and hygiene. The pioneering investigators in these fields have established a large body of knowledge that fuels ongoing research to this day. Knowing a little more about the history of nutrition and sports nutrition can help you to understand the role that nutrition plays in good health.

Food as Life

While the science of nutrition is still a relatively new discipline, the study of food and its effects on the body is not. The earliest recorded history shows that people have studied food since ancient times, investigating both how food nourishes the body and the *nutrients* supplied by food. Even in prehistoric times, people understood that the plants and animals around them were their sources of energy.

The earliest civilizations revolved around the need to find food, and later, the cultivation of it. We don't know for sure, but these early civilizations probably didn't spend a lot of time thinking about the different effects of the food they ate. They did understand that too much food could disrupt their normal bodily functions or make them sick. However, they also believed that such problems were sent by the gods as punishment for overindulging.

Foodie

Nutrients are nourishing substances that are essential to life.

The Hippocratic Method

One of the most influential early investigators of food and health was the Greek physician Hippocrates, who, in 400 B.C.E., advised his students to "Let thy food be thy medicine and thy medicine be thy food." Hippocrates believed that food was a potent medicine and that eating foods in their natural state could cure most illnesses. He said that bread could affect the body in different ways depending on how it was prepared (whether from pure flour or meal with bran, from winnowed or unwinnowed wheat, and so on), and believed that "each one of the substances of a man's diet acts upon his body and upon these changes his whole life depends."

The "father of modern medicine" advocated both exercise and proper nutrition as the keys to maintaining good health and preventing and reversing disease. Among his other recommendations were these:

♦ Dietary moderation—eating the proper amounts of food

♦ Adjusting food selection and amounts eaten based on the seasons of the year

♦ Eating regular meals—more than once a day

♦ Establishing and following a regular meal schedule

Eat It Up!

Hippocrates identified three types of nutrients necessary to sustain life: solids, beverages, and air. To maintain good health, these elements had to be in balance with the body's humors, or main fluids: blood, phlegm or lymph, yellow bile, and black bile. Disrupting this balance resulted in disease and bad temperament.

Hippocrates' observations were groundbreaking, as they were the first to suggest that the gods did not cause ill health. Instead, he saw disease for what it was: the result of poor dietary and exercise habits. The healing approach he developed, called the Hippocratic Method, would serve as the basis for medical practice for the next 17 centuries.

Galen's Guidelines for Good Health

Clarisimus Galenus, or Galen, another prominent Greek physician, expanded Hippocrates' observations into what we today would recognize as a holistic approach to good health. Throughout his life, he advised his patients to do the following:

- Eat right

- Drink the right beverages

- Get lots of fresh air

- Exercise regularly

- Get enough sleep

- Keep emotions under control

- Have a daily bowel movement

Galen, who lived from 129 c.e. to 201 c.e., is often noted as being one of the most famous physicians of all time. He was the physician to the gladiators, and based many of his observations on the benefits of exercise and nutrition on the care he gave them.

In his writings, Galen stressed the importance of exercise for all individuals—common person and gladiator alike—and suggested simple ways, such as playing with a small ball "which is so much a people's activity that even the poorest man is able to have the equipment," to make exercise easy and accessible for everyone as well as a part of everyday life.

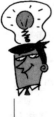 **Eat It Up!**

From their writings, we know that other ancient physicians understood that food could both cause disease and treat it. What they didn't know, however, was how exactly it did. They knew that night blindness could be cured by eating liver, and that eating beans caused bloating and flatulence, but they didn't know why. Those discoveries would come centuries later.

Galen also understood the importance of balance and advised his patients to practice every exercise in moderation. He disapproved of any activity that didn't use various body parts equally. Running, he felt, was a particularly poor choice, especially if it was done just to lose weight. He had similar distain for bodybuilding if the goal was merely to bulk up, and noted that the individuals who valued muscle mass over the "pursuit of excellence" often became "so weighted down that they have difficulty breathing."

Fueling Ancient Athletes

We also know from early writings that people understood that there was a link between food and athletic performance. Although we don't have a great deal to go on, there are both written and visual accounts of various nutritional strategies and training routines followed by ancient Greek and Roman athletes on the advice of their trainers. Since they lacked scientific knowledge, these ancient athletes and their coaches relied mostly on superstition, believing that certain foods would enhance performance or keep them well, while others would hamper their performance or cause them to get ill.

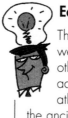

Eat It Up!

The first sports nutritionists were the physicians and other individuals who advised and trained the athletes who competed in the ancient Olympic Games.

Pythagoras, the noted Greek philosopher and mathematician, was also an athletic trainer. He is often credited for being the first person to train athletes on a meat diet, which he believed would help boxers and wrestlers build bulk and stamina. Other popular performance foods of the period included bread made from barley or raw wheat, porridges, meal (grain) cakes, dried figs, moist cheeses, honey, and wine.

The Olympics were abolished in 393 C.E., at about the same time that the Dark Ages began in Europe. During this period, scholarship and scientific inquiry ground to a halt in this part of the world. To the east, however, Islamic civilization was on the rise. Medicine played a central role in medieval Islam, and Islamic physicians and scholars continued the traditions of the Greeks and the Romans. They also preserved what was left of the written works of both civilizations. Many important scientific and medical texts, including those written by Galen and Hippocrates, were translated into Arabic for ease of use.

As the Dark Ages drew to a close, interest in science was revived in Europe. Those who were interested in matters of nutrition and exercise now had an even broader body of work to draw from, thanks to the contributions of physicians and scientists of the Islamic world.

The Modern Era of Nutritional Research

In modern times, one of the first discoveries related to the importance of nutrients in human health was made in the 1670s when a British physician named Thomas Sydenham observed that patients suffering from anemia regained their health when they drank iron filings mixed in wine. About 70 years after this discovery, James Lind, a British naval surgeon, tested a number of possible treatments on sailors who were suffering from scurvy. When their usual shipboard diet was exchanged for one that was laden with citrus fruits and cider, their symptoms subsided.

Other discoveries that linked certain foods to the prevention of physical problems included:

- Using iodine (found in sea vegetables and salt taken from areas rich with them) to treat goiter.

- Eating unmilled rice to prevent beriberi.

- Using fish oil to prevent rickets.

- Replacing a diet that relies on dishes made from corn with a more balanced diet to prevent pellagra.

With the exception of goiter and anemia, all of these diseases are related to vitamin deficiencies. A lack of vitamin C causes scurvy. Rice coatings, which are removed when rice is milled, contain vitamin B1, orthiamine, which prevents beriberi. Fish oil contains vitamin D. Pellagra results from eating a diet that lacks B3, or niacin.

How the Body Uses Food

While some scientists focused on learning more about the components of food that supported good health, others looked at the *physiology* of the body, or how the human body actually works. Part of their inquiry included studying how the body keeps going and what it needs to do so.

In the 1500s, Michelangelo compared the body's metabolic process to a "burning candle." In the late 1700s, Antoine Lavoisier, a French chemist, took Michelangelo's theory a step further. In 1789, along with his partner Pierre Laplace, Lavoisier conducted tests on guinea pigs and humans to demonstrate how the body gets its energy from food. His tests showed that the body uses oxygen to produce carbon dioxide and water, and that the amount of oxygen used corresponded to the amount of food that was consumed and the amount of physical activity that was being done.

Lavoisier also designed a tool called a calorimeter that measured the heat produced by the body from work and consumption of varying amounts and types of food. Today known as the "father of nutrition," Lavoisier also is famous for his statement, "Life is a chemical process."

Other physiological discoveries of the modern era included those made by:

♦ Robert Boyle, the "father of modern chemistry," who in the late 1600s conducted experiments that proved that oxygen was essential for combustion and respiration.

♦ Rene-Antoine Fercault de Reaumur, who conducted regurgitation experiments to prove that digestion was a chemical reaction and not a result of a mechanical process in the body.

♦ Archibald Vivian Hill, who studied muscle action, and especially how muscles produce heat. His research led to the discovery that muscular heat was produced by the passage of nerve impulses. For his efforts, he shared the 1922 Nobel Prize in Physiology or Medicine with another noted researcher in the area of physiology—Otto Fritz Meyerhof, who was honored for his discovery of the relationship of oxygen consumption and lactic acid metabolism in the muscles.

♦ Wilbur Olin Atwater, one of the founding fathers of modern nutritional science, who conducted a series of metabolic experiments that measured how the body used food for energy. In so doing, he determined the calorie values for a number of foods and developed calorie tables that are still in use today.

Foodie

Physiology is the branch of biology that deals with the internal workings of living things, including such functions as metabolism, respiration, and reproduction. **Metabolism** is the continuous and ongoing series of interrelated chemical reactions in the body that provide the energy and nutrients needed to sustain life.

By the beginning of the twentieth century, researchers had a pretty good idea of how the body worked, what it needed for fuel, and how it produced energy from food. They had also defined the chemical composition of protein, carbohydrate, and fat. Now it was time to find out exactly what it was about these foods that either supported or undermined good health.

Digging Into Food

It was in the twentieth century that most of the discoveries regarding nutrients took place. Scientists began to take a closer look at what food was actually made of. As they did, they isolated individual vitamins, minerals, amino acids, fatty acids, and other substances contained in food that would later define the basics of human nutrition.

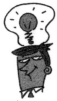

Eat It Up!

Experiments conducted on cattle feed led to the isolation of vitamin A. The B vitamins came soon after, along with Vitamin C. At the same time, researchers found that minute amounts of certain minerals contained in food and water were also dietary essentials.

Over time, improved transportation systems, food preservation techniques such as refrigeration, canning, and freezing, and nutrient-fortified foods lessened or eliminated many of the nutrient-deficiency diseases in the United States and in other industrialized countries. With these issues largely under control, nutrition scientists could now focus on the relationship between modern dietary patterns and chronic or deadly diseases like cancer, diabetes, high blood pressure, and other heart problems. Research in these areas continues to this day as scientists work to unlock more of the mysteries behind food and health, including what makes the body function and what we need to give it when those functions short-circuit.

The Evolution of Sports Nutrition

As previously mentioned, less research has been done on the nutritional needs of athletes over the years as there was no central force to drive such inquiry. After the ancient Olympics came to an end in the fourth century C.E., much less attention was paid to sport and athletics. There were some studies conducted on rowers and walkers during the nineteenth century, but these investigations fell far short of being a comprehensive body of work.

With the reestablishment of the modern Olympics in 1896, interest in performance nutrition began to build. Some studies were done during the years following the first modern games, but it wasn't until the 1936 Olympics in Berlin that a serious look at Olympian eating patterns was undertaken.

Performance Eating, Olympic Style

Several researchers studied the eating habits of the athletes at the Berlin games. From their writings, it was clear that while food choices varied a bit depending on the country and its nutritional traditions and beliefs, animal protein—specifically, red meat—played a significant role in the diets of athletes from many countries. Participants at the 1936 Games also chowed down on grains in the form of bread, pasta, rice, and cold and hot cereal. Vegetables, both cooked and raw, played a far lesser role—in fact, they were absent from a good number of training tables. Fruit, on the other hand, was a fairly common feature.

Probing the Food-Performance Connection

The eating habits of the athletes at the Berlin Olympics reflected a polyglot of nutritional beliefs that were based on superstitions and cultural traditions more than on sound science. In the years that followed, however, nutrition scientists and physiologists began to take a closer look at exactly how different foods could be used to fuel athletic performance and help athletes recover from their efforts. They also began to investigate the energy demands of individual sports and how food choices and eating patterns could be tailored to optimize the performance of the athletes who competed in them.

Dawn Says

The body needs regular doses of fuel to run like it's supposed to. However, many people skip meals and wait until they have little energy before they refuel. I like to compare bodies to coal-burning trains. The engineers on those old trains didn't wait until the last ember died to stoke the fire. If they had, the trains would have come to a halt. Nor did they get overzealous and fill the coal bin to the very top. Doing so would have smothered the fire, producing little or no energy. Instead, they kept the fires going at a constant level, and regularly added just enough fuel to keep things running smoothly. It's the same thing when you're fueling your body.

Sports Nutrition Today

All of the probing and poking around in the realms of nutrition and physiology has resulted in a science that combines the best knowledge from both arenas. Good nutrition is essential to good health, no matter who you are. Sports nutrition takes the principles of good nutrition a step further. It looks at what you do with your body, and tailors both the things you eat and when you eat them to enhance your activities. It takes into account the big picture—all your workouts, practices, classes, competitions—whatever it is you like to do.

Sports nutrition also takes into account the various nutritional needs of different sports. If you're a weight lifter, you're going to eat differently than an ice skater would. If you're a beginning runner training for your first 10k, your nutritional needs will be different than those of an experienced marathon runner.

Tailoring nutrition to activities can do amazing things for athletes of all shapes, sizes, and persuasions. It can do the following:

- Maximize concentration
- Minimize fatigue
- Reduce errors
- Attain and maintain ideal body composition
- Decrease the use of harmful supplements and illegal substances used to "get up" for the game
- Optimize your time in the gym
- Minimize recovery time

Eat It Up!

Sports nutrition focuses on three main factors that support good health and optimal exercise performance: choosing the appropriate food and fluids, timing their intake to enhance performance and recovery, and using the appropriate supplements.

Sports nutrition gives "eating to live" a whole new meaning. Nutrition is just nutrition. Sports nutrition will get you to where you want to go.

The Least You Need to Know

- The sciences of nutrition and sports nutrition are relatively new. The term nutrition was unknown until the late 1800s. Sports nutrition was introduced in the middle of the twentieth century.
- The earliest sports nutritionists were the physicians and other individuals who helped train the athletes who competed in the ancient Olympic Games.
- Following a good sports nutrition program can enhance athletic performance and decrease injuries.
- Sports nutrition focuses on three main factors that support optimal health and exercise performance: appropriate food and fluid selection, timing their intake to enhance performance and recovery, and appropriate supplementation.

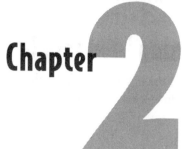

Chapter 2

Fueling Up

In This Chapter

- ◆ Where we get our energy
- ◆ What our bodies do with what we eat
- ◆ Understanding metabolism
- ◆ All about ATP

Everyone knows that eating is essential to life, but many people don't know what their bodies actually do with the nutrients that they put into them. We know that those burgers and salads that we eat keep us going, but how?

No matter who you are, your body works in basically the same way. In this chapter, we'll explore how your body uses the food you feed it and why it's important for active people of all types to feed their bodies right.

You'll see some biological and chemical terms in this chapter, which might make it a little slow going if you're rusty when it comes to these sciences. We'll make it as easy to understand as we can.

Turning Food Into Energy

Human beings are basically big energy machines. We take in energy and we output energy. The energy exchange process in our body is called *metabolism*.

There are two types of metabolism:

Foodie

Metabolism is the process of chemical digestion and its related reactions that provide the energy and nutrients needed to sustain life.

♦ Catabolism, or destructive metabolism. In catabolism, large organic molecules are broken down into smaller molecules. As they are broken down, they release energy.

♦ Anabolism, or constructive metabolism. In anabolism, small molecules are assembled into large molecules. This requires the input of energy.

These breaking-down and building-up processes go on nonstop in the body, which means we are always using energy in some way. Respiration, heart function, and new cell formation are examples of processes that use this kind of energy. Some people think that after 8 P.M. at night or when they go to bed this process stops. If this were true, however, people would only live for a day. Metabolism, or energy, enables our involuntary physiological mechanisms to operate around the clock.

In plants, metabolism takes the form of photosynthesis, which is the building of sugars. This is what plants, algae, and some bacteria do to feed themselves. They use the power of the sun to help them combine carbon dioxide and water to make glucose and oxygen gas.

Since humans depend on outside sources of nutrients—food—to meet their energy needs, the metabolic process is a little different. Here's what it entails:

Eat It Up!

All living things, including humans, get their energy from plants and from other living things that eat plants. Ultimately, all of our energy comes from plants, whether we eat them directly or eat animals that feed on plants.

♦ First, food—carbohydrate, fat, and protein— is ingested.

♦ The body then uses various enzymes and water to convert food to chemicals that the body can use, such as sugars, amino acids, fatty acids, and so on.

♦ These chemicals are absorbed into the body and transported to the cells, where they are absorbed.

Once the molecules make it into the cells, they are again broken down into even simpler molecules. From here, they might serve as the building blocks for all sorts of cellular activities. Or they might be broken down again. As they are, they eventually turn back into inorganic molecules such as carbon dioxide, water, and ammonia.

The main source of energy in the cells is a molecule called adenosine triphosphate, or ATP. As you'll see in a minute, this is one important little piece of matter.

Understanding ATP

ATP, or adenosine triphosphate, is a special molecule—technically, an adenine nucleotide bound to three phosphates—that your body creates to store and use energy. ATP is made by the mitochondria of the cells and is made when and where the cells need it. ATP provides energy for most of the energy-consuming activities of the cell, including the construction of proteins from amino acids, the assembly of nucleotides (a type of chemical compound) into DNA and RNA, and carbohydate and fat synthesis. Among other things, ATP also does the following:

- Moves molecules and ions into and out of cell membranes through a process called active transport

- Assists nerve impulses

- Helps the cells maintain their volume

ATP is also the primary energy-producing molecule that your body uses for muscle contraction. The process that turns ATP into energy is pretty complicated, but basically, when a cell needs energy, it breaks apart the ATP molecule. As ATP breaks apart, it releases energy by bonding with water. At the same time, it loses a phosphate atom and turns into adenosine diphosphate (ADP).

The body can only make enough ATP to last for a few minutes at rest. As the work of the muscle increases, more ATP is consumed, and it leaves the body at a faster rate. In order for the muscle to keep working, ATP must be replaced.

ATP production is so important to the body that it has three different energy systems that create it—the phosphagen system, the glycogen-lactic system, and the aerobic-respiration system. The systems all work together to create energy transfer during exercise, and overlap during the process depending on how long and how hard you're working out. Your fitness level and oxygen uptake (your body's ability to use oxygen efficiently) will also determine when each system kicks in. As the intensity levels of your workout fluctuate, your body will switch between all three systems.

As an example, let's say you're going to row a 2,000-meter race. During the first few seconds after you start, your muscle cells will burn off any ATP that they already contain. Then, the phosphagen system kicks in and supplies energy for the next eight to ten seconds. Since your activity is lasting longer than this, the glycogen-lactic acid system kicks in for the next three minutes or so. Finally, the aerobic-respiration system kicks in for the remaining duration of your event.

The Phosphagen Energy System

Muscle cells are limited in the amount of ATP they have at their immediate disposal because the body can only make so much of it at one time. When the body needs to replenish ATP levels quickly, it takes a replacement phosphate atom from another molecule called creatine phosphate (CP), which it uses to replenish the ADP molecule. Presto! A new ATP molecule, courtesy of the phosphagen energy system.

Eat It Up!

The phosphagen system gets its name from the creatine phosphate atom it uses to replace the missing phosphate atom. Its system is considered anaerobic, meaning that it doesn't need oxygen to work. For this reason, it is sometimes called the "immediate energy system."

The phosphagen energy system is used during rapid, high-intensity activities that require a short burst of power, such as sprints, lifting heavy weights, jumping, throwing, and diving, when the muscles aren't supplied by oxygen. Because it lacks oxygen, this energy system can only provide enough energy to sustain these activities for bursts of time—no more than five to ten seconds.

The Glycogen-Lactic Energy System

This energy system uses the glycogen molecules—or carbohydrate stores—that are deposited in the muscles from food metabolism. It comes into play during activities that are moderate to high in intensity and medium in length, such as medium-distance runs and swims. When the muscles need energy, they convert glycogen into glucose, and then into a substance called pyruvate. From here, the pyruvate enters the mitochondria of the cells, where it helps make more ATP.

The glycogen-lactic energy system is also called the glycolytic energy system, or simply glycolysis. For ease, we'll refer to it as the glycolytic energy system from here on.

The glycolytic energy system, like the phosphagen system, is also anaerobic. However, it can also take place if oxygen is present. This type of glycolytic energy is called "aerobic" because it uses oxygen. When glycolysis takes place where there isn't enough oxygen, it creates lactic acid, which further breaks down to lactate and hydrogen ions.

Dawn Says
For many years, lactic acid, the byproduct of anaerobic glycolysis, was believed to be the substance that makes your muscles hurt. We now know that it is the accumulation of hydrogen ions—another byproduct of lactic acid breakdown—that is primarily responsible for muscle pain. Lactic acid actually plays a positive role in the metabolic process. When enough oxygen is present, the body converts it back into pyruvate, which it then uses for making more energy.

Aerobic Respiration

This energy system takes place in the mitochondria of the cells when there is enough oxygen to meet the demands of the activity. For this reason, it is sometimes called the aerobic energy system or mitochondrial respiration. It kicks in when exercise continues beyond several minutes, as it does during sports like rowing, distance running or swimming, or cross-country skiing. To meet the energy needs of the muscles, the body supplies them with oxygen. This allows glucose to be completely broken down into carbon dioxide and water, which results in even more energy release, or ATP production. Glycogen isn't the only thing that can fuel aerobic respiration, which is why this energy system can keep going for hours if necessary. Fatty acids from the body's fat reserves and muscles can also be used. If absolutely necessary, the body will even break down proteins into amino acids and use it to make ATP, although it doesn't like to do this and will only do it in extreme situations.

Dawn Says
In order to tap into your fat stores efficiently, oxygen must be present. This is why people who are trying to decrease body-fat levels are advised to add cardio workouts to their training sessions.

As much as we'd like to burn more fat as fuel, it simply won't happen. Here's why:

♦ It takes too long to convert during intense activity.

♦ The body needs more oxygen to burn it.

♦ Lactic acid hinders the utilization of fat. The less oxygen available, the more the body relies on glucose. Because the intensity is high, more pyruvate is converted into lactic acid, which then slows the oxygen supply needed to use fat as fuel.

However, this doesn't mean that you should avoid high-intensity workouts when trying to lose body fat. If you work out at higher intensities, you'll actually burn more fat during a workout. A workout at high intensity lasting only 30 minutes will burn more fat than one for 45 minutes at a moderate intensity. Also remember that when working out you are burning energy (calories). After you work out, your body will then pull stored fat out of storage to meet your energy needs.

When compared to the other energy systems, aerobic respiration and the aerobic form of glycolytic energy system produce and activate energy much more slowly. Because of this, these slower systems can continue to supply ATP for several hours or longer, as long as nutrients are available.

The following chart compares the three energy systems. Note how large a role carbohydrates play. In fact, even during light to moderate exercise, carbohydrates supply approximately 40 to 60 percent of your total energy. Fat comes next, and protein comes last, generally comprising less than 10 percent of the energy required for exercise.

Energy System	Phosphagen	Glycolytic (anaerobic)	Aerobic Respiration
Duration	Less than 10 secs.	10 secs. to 3 min.	Greater than 3 min.
Intensity	Very high to high	High to mod.	Moderate to low
Fuel source	Primarily CP	Carbohydrates in the form of glucose and stored glucose	Carbohydrates (primarily), then fat, then protein
Oxygen needed	No	No	Yes
Events	Sprints, power lifting, jumping, diving	Middle-distance run, 50m swim	Long-distance events—runs, swims, rowing, etc.

When talking about how the body uses its energy stores to fuel performance, these three energy systems are often simply referred to as anaerobic pathways and aerobic pathways. As a reminder, the phosphagen energy system is entirely anaerobic; the glycolytic energy system can be both anaerobic and aerobic; and the aerobic respiration system is completely aerobic.

Whenever we start exercising, we mainly use glucose as our fuel source and the anaerobic pathway to create energy. Once we warm up and our heart starts pumping faster (in about 20 minutes or so), oxygen-enriched (aerobic) blood supplies our muscles. At this point, the body starts to use fatty acids, some glucose, and a very small amount of protein in the form of amino acids.

The Shape You're In

As previously mentioned, your fitness level and oxygen uptake level—that is, how well your muscles take oxygen out of the blood and into the muscle cells—will also determine what fuel sources your body uses during exercise. Oxygen uptake, or VO_2 max, is genetically predetermined to a large extent, but you can improve it with training. Untrained people with lower oxygen uptake levels tend to build lactic acid faster because their muscles don't get enough oxygen when they exercise. The more lactic acid builds up, the less fat you burn.

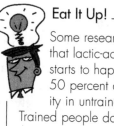

Eat It Up!

Some research suggests that lactic-acid buildup starts to happen at around 50 percent aerobic capacity in untrained individuals. Trained people don't get it until they're up to about 70 percent of their aerobic capacity. This lets them use more fat and spare their glycogen stores.

When you're well trained and have a higher aerobic capacity, your muscles are able to use more oxygen. Being in shape also increases the glycogen-storing capacity of the muscles, which makes recovery after exercise easier.

Stoking Your Body's Energy Burners

Now that you know more about how your body uses the food you eat for fuel, let's take a quick look at the fuel requirements for short, intermediate, and long-term sports. We will go into this in more depth in later chapters.

Fueling for Short-Term Sports

Since these sports last only up to four minutes, and your energy source is glucose/glycogen, having optimal levels of glycogen in the body is imperative.

Creatine supplementation may be of benefit for these athletes since creatine phosphate also helps supply energy in high demand over a short time period. To spare the body's glycogen stores, training before the day of the event should be little to none, and your warm-up the day of the event should not be at intermittent high intervals. If you are competing several times during the day, pre- and post-event snacks or meals will help you keep your carbohydrate stores their fullest for the next time you compete.

Fueling for Intermediate-Term Sports

These sports last anywhere from four to nine minutes, and may be longer. They use glucose/glycogen for their main energy source. Due to their high intensity and short duration, they don't use fat for energy.

For optimal performance, tapering training and increasing carbohydrates two to three days prior to competition is recommended for optimal glycogen storage. The day of the event, you will use your glycogen stores, so you'll need to plan for hydrating and refueling during the day.

Fueling for Long-Term Sports

These activities last longer than 90 minutes of continuous aerobic activity. Again, having optimal levels of muscle glycogen is critical for these sports. Well-trained athletes actually store more glycogen than the untrained. You can improve your glycogen stores by:

◆ Following a high-carbohydrate eating program for the week before the event.

◆ Decreasing your workouts.

◆ Taking a couple of days off prior to your event.

Proper hydration and taking in 30 to 60 grams of carbohydrates every hour during competition will help keep energy supply at optimal levels.

Foods for Fuel

To complete our look at how the body uses fuel for energy, let's take a few minutes for a quick survey of the foods it uses. We'll get into much more detail on all of them in Part 2.

Carbohydrates

As you now know, carbohydrates are vital for optimal performance. It is important to have enough carbohydrates, but it is also important to properly time your intake of them. The body can only store approximately 500 to 600 grams of carbohydrates in the liver and muscle. Since we use carbohydrates for fuel, the body will also recover faster if you eat some within two hours after your workout. Also, if you mix carbohydrates with a little protein after a meal, your body will absorb even more carbohydrates.

Carbohydrates are found in the following foods. All measurements are in grams. The amounts given are based on one serving of each food. For more information on serving sizes, turn to Chapter 5.

Food	Carbs	Protein	Fat
Grains	15	3	0–1
Fruit	15	0	0
Vegetables	5	3	0
Dairy	12	8	0–5
Meat	0	7	0–5

You should consume anywhere from 45 to 70 percent of carbohydrates a day, depending on how many calories you take in a day and on your sport. To know what your level should be, calculate your needs based on 6 to 10 grams per kg (2.2 lbs) of body weight. Here is an example:

You weigh 175 pounds

175/2.2kg = 80 kg

80 kg × 6 = 420 grams of carbohydrates a day

Dawn Says

Carbohydrate loading can be very useful in long-distance sports lasting longer than 90 minutes. Research shows that using this method can increase your carbohydrate stores (glycogen) by 50 to 100 percent. However, you need to be well trained before this can work. Endurance training stimulates the synthesis of muscle glycogen. This technique is not good for intermediate or short-term distances. This amount of carbs can make you feel heavy at first. This is due to the amount of water you store with the carbs—one glucose molecule stored in muscle brings with it three molecules of water. Since the activity lasts so long, this heaviness subsides. In shorter time spans, this heaviness can negatively affect your performance. Your workouts must decrease significantly for a week, especially three days prior, or this technique will not work.

Protein

Protein does not like to be used as fuel. Instead, it likes to be used to build, maintain, and repair tissues. If you fuel yourself properly, the maximum amount of energy from protein that your body will use is 5 percent. If you are running low on carbs and your exercise is long in duration, your body will use up to 10 percent protein for energy.

If your intake of calories on a daily basis is low, well below the energy you need for maintenance, your body will use even more protein.

When you work out, your body increases the amount of epinephrine in your system and decreases insulin levels. This may be the reason why during exercise there is more protein breakdown instead of protein building. Many supplements claim they can help minimize protein breakdown. However, the positive outweighs the negative here, as exercise also increases the efficiency of protein building that happens after a workout and during recovery.

Dawn Says

The recommended daily amount of protein is 0.8 gram per kg of body weight. I personally believe that this level is too low for anyone. I start people out at 1.0 gram per kg of body weight if they're inactive. If you are active, your protein requirement will range from between 1.2 grams to 1.8 grams per kg of body weight. People who compete in endurance sports/long distance sports should eat around 1.2 grams per kg; body builders should be around 1.8 grams per kg.

The body can only absorb a certain amount of protein every three to four hours, so it is important to have protein with your meals and snacks to get it all in. Women usually absorb from 7 to 20 grams of protein and men usually absorb 14 to 30 grams of protein every 3 to 4 hours.

When I create individual menus for my clients, I first figure out their protein needs and then divide this number by how many meals and snacks I want them to have in a day. Depending on their starting calorie needs, their protein intake may be higher, but as they continue training and they burn more energy I then add more carbohydrates and fat, since they are already at optimal protein levels.

Protein intake should not exceed 20 to 30 percent of your total daily calories. Protein, as you now know, is not a main source of energy. High-protein diets will use up your glycogen stores over time and make you feel tired and sluggish. Using protein as the main fuel for energy can result in injuries, decreased muscle mass, and poor performance.

Fat

Fat supplies anywhere from 20 to 30 percent of total intake a day, depending on your sport. Eating more than these levels can impair your intake of other important nutrients, and it won't improve your performance, even if you compete in sports that require some fat for energy. Most athletes store enough fat anyway, so additional fat intake above these levels isn't needed.

The Least You Need to Know

♦ The energy exchange process in both plants and animals is called metabolism.

♦ ATP is also the primary energy-producing molecule that your body uses for muscle contraction.

♦ The body has three different energy systems that kick in at different times and produce ATP in different ways.

♦ The body can absorb only a certain amount of protein every 3 to 4 hours—women usually absorb from 7 to 20 grams of protein, men usually absorb 14 to 30 grams.

♦ Eating more protein will not boost your energy. In fact, it can do exactly the opposite.

Performance Eating

In This Chapter

- ◆ How to keep your internal engine running smoothly
- ◆ The importance of eating enough calories
- ◆ Visual cues for portion control
- ◆ Sample eating plans for optimal performance

Now that you know how your body uses food as fuel, it's time to take a closer look at how to use the food you eat to power your physical activity. No matter who you are or what kind of shape you're in, eating the right food and eating it at the right times can make a big difference in what you do and how you feel while you're doing it.

Some people think that the principles of sports nutrition only apply to athletes who participate in competitive sports, either at the amateur or professional level, but nothing could be further from the truth. Active people come in all shapes and sizes. They may enjoy competitive sports, or they may not. Someone who exercises regularly can benefit just as much from knowing how to eat to fuel his or her activity as the football player who takes the field every Sunday.

There's an athlete inside of everyone. The principles of sports nutrition bring out that athlete and help all active people reach their individual goals.

Different People, Different Goals

We often think of athletes as these exalted individuals who pretty much came out of the womb trained to peak perfection, but the truth is that they had to start at the beginning just like everyone else. While they may be blessed with some genetic attributes that set them apart from the rest of us, they're not much different from you and me. They've just decided, for a variety of reasons, to reach for some lofty goals when it comes to what they do with their bodies, and they use sports nutrition to help them get there.

What are your goals? Do you want to better your time for the half-mile, train for a regional karate meet, decrease your body fat, better your cardiovascular health? Or maybe you're interested in taking your own fitness level up a notch and competing for the first time in your favorite event. Whatever your goal, the following nutritional guidelines, which apply to everyone regardless of activity or fitness level, are the basics for helping you get there.

Eat Regular Meals

Don't skip meals, and especially don't pass by breakfast and lunch. By incorporating breakfast into your daily routine, you get your engines going. It's like starting your car on a cold morning. You turn over the engine and you let it warm up before you drive off. When you're ready to leave, your car is warm and ready to go. Breakfast is the same thing. By fueling your body in the morning, you're warming up your muscles and brain cells to function at their best.

Eat It Up!

You'll burn 5 to 10 percent more energy (calories) if you include breakfast and lunch in your everyday eating pattern. If you don't like to eat breakfast or your stomach is a bit uneasy in the morning, try drinking a liquid meal replacement instead. There are many types that are fast and easy to digest.

If you think that eating breakfast will make you hungrier, well, you're right. Do you expect your car to keep going without gas after you've driven it around for awhile? Do you expect that a coal-fueled train doesn't have to be consistently restoked? Eating gets your engine started, too, and once it's up and running it needs to be fed on a regular basis. Getting hungry is good, it's normal. Your body is telling you it needs more energy—more food.

Eat Often

The best way to keep your engine going the way it should is to eat every three to four hours. This gives your body a constant stream of energy throughout the day. It also helps prevent the ups and downs in energy you might get, especially in the mid-morning or mid-afternoon. By eating frequent meals, you are less likely to get really hungry and overeat. You're also less likely to just grab anything you can (usually foods that are highly processed, high in sugar, high in fat, and low in nutrients) to quash your hunger pains.

Most people who eat every three to four hours do so by eating three large meals and two snacks a day. Depending on your daily routine and workouts, you may need to eat three meals a day plus three snacks. If eating that many times a day is just too hard or too time-consuming, you must have a minimum of three meals a day. By eating frequently, your body is able to process and assimilate the nutrients more efficiently, which leads to more calories being burned and less being turned into fat.

Eat Enough

Make sure you are taking in enough energy. Many people believe that less is better, but if you don't take in enough energy, you'll burn muscle instead of fat. Muscles require more fuel to work, so the more muscle we have, the more energy we need.

I've talked to many people, both clients and not, who believe that they don't have to eat very much. Here's why: People tend to believe that they need only a certain amount of energy to function every day. However, instead of calculating what their energy needs are, they seemingly pluck a number out of the air. Unfortunately, this number is often way too low.

As an example, I have worked with a 150-pound female basketball player who was at 18 percent body fat when I met her. She burned 3,000 calories a day, but believed that less was better and ate only 1,800 calories a day. She maintained her weight at this level of caloric intake. Her college basketball career showed a history of injuries toward the middle of the season and a feeling of sluggishness toward the end of the season. So why wasn't her weight and body fat lower if she was taking in fewer calories than she was burning (it takes 3,500 calories to lose a pound of fat)? By her calculations, she was supposed to be losing 2.4 pounds a week, but she was maintaining her weight. What happened was this: Her metabolism adjusted to her low intake.

Your metabolism begins to adjust within two to three weeks from the time you start varying your calories. This is why some people lose weight quickly at first. However, as the months go by, it becomes more difficult. The body believes it needs to protect itself, so it slows down the amount of weight loss and starts to equal out what you burn to what you eat. Plus, when you decrease your intake by too much too soon, your body will use muscle for energy and retain the fat. In this athlete's case, her weight stayed the same but her body fat increased to 20 percent by the end of the season. This could have been the main reason she was getting injured and feeling sluggish.

When I started working with her in the preseason the following year, we got her energy intake up to around 3,000 calories a day. As her intake went up, her body weight went down 2 pounds and her body fat decreased to 16 percent. She finished the season with almost the same numbers. She sustained her energy, had only one ankle sprain, but recovered quickly, and had her best stats ever.

The moral of the story? Making sure we take in the proper amount of nutrients is very important for overall performance.

Keep Track of Your Intake

Unless your memory is really good, it's difficult to remember everything you eat. When you're eating for optimal nutrition, it's important that you keep a daily food record. Turn to Chapter 4 for more on this, as well as a chart to assist your tracking efforts.

Balance Your Macronutrients

Eat a mix of foods at each meal. Always try to have a mix of carbohydrates, protein, and fat. This will ensure that you get the nutrients you need and also get a constant amount of energy. Carbohydrates tend to be absorbed into the bloodstream more quickly than protein and fat, and certain kinds of carbohydrates are absorbed faster than others. By mixing your foods—eating faster-absorbing foods with foods that don't get into the bloodstream as fast—you can create a more constant energy stream. Having this constant stream of energy also helps decrease body fat, which you can read more about in Chapter 23. Plus, when you eat a mixture of foods, you get a variety of important nutrients.

Eat Lots of Fruit and Vegetables

The government recommends a total of five fruits and vegetables a day for most people, but a much better intake level is four of each every day. Fruits and vegetables are a good source of vitamins, fiber, water, and energy. The nutrients in fruits and vegetables can help with wound recovery, and help prevent oxidative stress, which damages cells, vessel walls, and even the nucleus of a cell. This is important for preventing flu, colds, and other ailments, and for recovering from workouts.

Minimize Empty Calories

It isn't called junk food for nothing! Chips, candy, sweets, fast food, fried food, and processed food are generally high in calories and/or fat, and low in nutrients. Most Americans consume at least two of these items a day, if not more. Home-cooked, wholesome meals are becoming a thing of the past unless we do something about it.

Watch Portion Sizes

One of the reasons obesity is on the rise is that our portion sizes are as well. What's more, it's not just our fast-food habits that are increasing our need for bigger belts. Researchers have found an astonishing amount of portion distortion going on in the home as well. After too many years of gulping down gargantuan soft drinks and supersized meals, many people simply don't know what normal portion sizes look like.

Now, we know how much of a pain it is to have to measure out portions. No one likes to do it, which is why people who follow diets that require them to measure out everything they eat usually fail at them. Some dietitians now teach their clients to learn how to judge portion sizes visually by comparing a standard portion to an everyday object. While it's not as exact as using measuring spoons, cups, and scales, it's a heck of a lot easier.

Here are some examples:

- A deck of cards = 3 ounces of meat or a small chicken breast
- Four dice = 1 ounce of cubed hard cheese
- A clenched fist = $\frac{1}{2}$ cup of pasta
- A baseball = 1 cup of raw vegetables

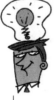

Eat It Up!

Did you know that if you ordered a combo meal from McDonald's in the 1960s you would have received a hamburger, small fries, and a medium drink—pretty similar to a kiddie meal today! People tend to eat very large portions today. If you're not sure about how much 1 cup or 1 ounce of food looks like, start to measure and weigh your food for one week. You'll be surprised at how much—or how little—you're actually eating.

Another good way to rein in your portion sizes is to measure your food for one week. Don't change the portions you would normally eat, just load them into measuring cups or spoons before you eat them. Keep a running record as you do on a notepad or index card. Total everything at the end of each day or at the end of the week and then compare the number of portions you've eaten to the recommended amounts. If you're not sure what these are, turn to Chapter 6 for more information.

Drink Plenty of Fluids

It's hard to overemphasize the importance of proper hydration, and it's not just athletes who need to ensure that their bodies contain enough fluid. Our body weight is composed of 40 to 70 percent water. Every reaction that happens in the body involves water in one way or another. Muscle building, muscle breakdown, and muscle contraction are all affected by the levels of water within the body.

Adequate hydration is essential for everyone, and it's especially important if you're active. If you're working out hard, you're going to perspire. Sweat a lot and you'll lose a lot of weight as well. For every pound of weight you lose when working out, you need 16 ounces of fluid to begin the rehydration process. Early fatigue is a sign of dehydration, and thirst is not a good indicator of fluid needs, as the sensation doesn't kick in until you're already dehydrated. People who work out, and athletes especially, need to be adequately hydrated before, during, and after practice and competition to achieve optimal performance.

In the chapters that follow, you'll find tons of information that will help you put the principles in this chapter into practice to build your own nutritional program.

Fueling Your Activities

Up to now you've been reading about the theories of sports nutrition. Now let's take a look at how they work in the real world. What follows is a series of food plans reflecting the different nutritional and hydration needs related to various activities of different lengths and intensities. As you go through them, you'll notice that they differ when it comes to how nutrients are balanced—the plan for short-term events, for example, is heavier in carbohydrates than the ones for longer events. As you read in Chapter 2, these activities call for a burst of energy that's fueled by glucose or glycogen provided by carbohydrates. To do them well, your body needs to have this fuel readily available.

These food plans are meant to be examples, not gospel. They're based on the energy and nutrient needs of a 150-pound female with 30 percent body fat eating 2,200 calories a day (you'll find adjustments for higher calorie levels as well). As such, they won't fit your needs exactly, or anyone else's for that matter, as everyone's needs are different. But they illustrate the importance of timing your meals to make sure your fuel levels are where they should be. Doing so will ensure that you have the energy you need when you're participating in your chosen activities, regardless of what they are. If you are exhausted after a meet or a practice, chances are it's the lack of fluid and nutrients that makes you feel this way.

The other thing to keep an eye out for is how the nutrients are balanced through the course of the day. For example, each food plan reflects a late-afternoon workout. Notice how the meals eaten before that workout are lower in calories and contain less protein and fat. Fat slows down the amount of oxygen to your muscles up to two hours after you ingest it. When you're working out, you want to make sure that you can give your muscles as much oxygen as possible. So, out with the fat and the protein, and in with the carbs! The meal after the workout contains a good balance of carbohydrates and protein to assist in recovery and to help build back muscle that may have been lost.

Fueling for Short-Term Events

Short-term events include activities such as sprints, short-distance swimming, body building, short-distance cycling, and so on. These activities only last up to about four minutes, which means your energy source comes from glucose or glycogen.

Nutrient Balance: 60 percent carbohydrates

15–25 percent fat

15–25 percent protein

With these events, it is extremely important to be well fueled and well hydrated. If you do any of them competitively, what you eat prior to the day is also part of the plan. Since these sports only last up to four minutes, your energy source will be glucose/glycogen, which means that having optimal levels is imperative.

Menu for Short-Term Events

The following menus are based on a 60-20-20 balance of carbohydrates, fat, and protein.

Breakfast (7 A.M. – 8 A.M.)

1 cup oatmeal/dry/rolled oats	4 grains
16 oz. skim milk	2 dairy
½ cup dried fruit	1 fruit
1 TB. Flax Mill (flaxseeds)	1 healthy fat

Lunch (11 A.M. – 12 P.M.)

4 slices whole wheat bread (Brownberry brand is good)	4 grains
2 oz. lean turkey	2 proteins
2 tsp. mustard	extra
1 tomato, sliced	1 vegetable
2 oranges	2 fruits

Snack (3 P.M. – 4 P.M.)

1 low-fat yogurt	1 dairy
1/2 cup Grape Nuts	2 grain
8 oz. skim milk	1 dairy
2 1/2 cups fresh strawberries	2 fruits

5 P.M. – 6 P.M.

Workout. Drink 24 to 32 ounces of water (the goal is not to lose any weight during this time). Also drink 16 to 20 ounces of Gatorade or eat one fruit for energy. After workout, drink 24 ounces of water per pound lost—hopefully this won't be necessary.

Dinner (7 P.M.)

2 oz. grilled teriyaki chicken	2 proteins
3 cups mixed greens and vegetables	3 vegetables
1 small whole-grain roll	1 grain
1/2 avocado (if fat intake is low)	2 healthy fats
2 TB. lite Caesar dressing	1 healthy fat

If you want an evening snack, take an item from breakfast or lunch and move it to 9 to 10 P.M.

To boost calories to 2,400, add the following:

3 grains

1.5 proteins

1 fruit

1 vegetable

To boost calories to 2,700, add the following:

6 grains

3 proteins

2 fruits

2 vegetables

0–1 fat

To boost calories to 3,000, add the following:

9 grains

6 proteins

3 fruits

3 vegetables

0–2 fats

Fueling for Intermediate-Length Events

These are sports such as a mile run, gymnastics, wrestling, rowing, skating, and middle-distance swimming that last anywhere from four to nine minutes and maybe longer. They also use glucose/glycogen for their main energy source. Due to the high intensity and short duration, fat fuel is not used for energy.

Menu for Intermediate-Length Events

Nutrient balance: 55–60 percent carbohydrates

15–20 percent fat

15–25 percent protein

The following menus are based on 55-20-25 balance of carbs, fat, and protein.

Total servings from each food group:

8 grains

8 protein (1 serving = 1 ounce of meat)

5 fruits

4 milk

5 vegetables

0–2.5 fat—This varies if you drink 2 percent or higher milk, eat regular cheese, more than one egg yolk per three egg whites, or if the meat products you choose are higher than 3 grams of fat per ounce. For each time you choose higher fat items, subtract one fat serving. Try to choose your fat choices from unsaturated fats.

Breakfast (7 A.M. – 8 A.M.)

1 cup oatmeal/dry/rolled oats	4 grains
16 oz. skim milk	2 dairy
¹/₂ cup dried fruit	1 fruit
1 TB. Flax Mill (flaxseed oil)	1 healthy fat

Lunch (11 A.M. – 12 P.M.)

2 slices whole grain bread	2 grains
4 oz. lean turkey	4 proteins
2 tsp. mustard	extra
2 tomatoes, sliced	2 vegetables
1 orange	1 fruit

Snack (3 P.M. – 4 P.M.)

1 low-fat yogurt	1 dairy
¹/₂ cup Grape Nuts	1 grain
8 oz. skim milk	1 dairy
2¹/₂ cups fresh strawberries	2 fruits

5 P.M. – 6 P.M.

Workout. Drink 24 to 32 ounces of water.

6 P.M.

Drink 24 ounces of water per pound of fluid lost.

Drink 16 to 20 ounces of Gatorade or eat one fruit

Dinner (7 P.M.)

4 oz. grilled teriyaki chicken	4 proteins
3 cups mixed greens and vegetables	3 vegetables
1 small whole wheat roll	1 grain
$\frac{1}{8}$ avocado (if fat intake is low)	1 healthy fat
1 TB. lite Caesar dressing	$\frac{1}{2}$ healthy fat

For 2,400 calories, add the following:

2 grains

1 proteins

0 fruit

2 dairy

1 vegetable

0–0.5 fat

For 2,700 calories, add the following:

4 grains

2 proteins

1 fruit

3 dairy

3 vegetables

0–1 fat

For 3,000 calories, add the following:

> 5 grains
>
> 5 proteins
>
> 2 fruits
>
> 3 milk
>
> 0–1.5 fats

Dawn Says

If you compete in intermediate-term sports, you'll want to taper on your training and increase your carbohydrates two to three days prior to competition for optimal glycogen storage. On the day of the event, your body will use your glycogen stores, so you'll have to replenish them during the day to keep from getting fatigued.

Long-Distance Activities

These activities last for more than 10 minutes and include long-distance running, swimming, cycling, football, volleyball, baseball, and basketball.

> Nutrient balance: 60–70 percent carbohydrates
>
> 20–30 percent fat
>
> 10–15 percent protein

The following eating plan uses a 65-20-15 ratio of carbs, fat, and protein.

Total servings from each food group:

> 10 grains
>
> 3 proteins (1 serving of protein is 1 ounce of meat)
>
> 8 fruits
>
> 2 dairy
>
> 6 vegetables
>
> 0–4 fat (As above, added fat is based on your fat intake from other foods. Each time you choose a higher fat item, subtract one fat serving from your total.)

Breakfast (7 A.M. – 8 A.M.)

1 cup oatmeal/dry/rolled oats	4 grains
8 oz. skim milk	1 dairy
½ dried fruit	1 fruit
1 TB. Flax Mill	1 healthy fat

Lunch (11 A.M. – 12 P.M.)

2 slices whole grain bread	2 grains
1 oz. lean turkey	1 protein
2 tsp. mustard	extra
2 tomatoes, sliced	2 vegetables
1 orange	1 fruit

Snack (3 P.M. – 4 P.M.)

1 low-fat yogurt	1 dairy
½ cup Grape Nuts	1 grain
2½ cups fresh strawberries	2 fruits
1 cup baby carrots	1 vegetable

Workout (5 P.M. – 6 P.M.)

Drink 24 to 32 ounces of water. After workout, drink 24 ounces of water per pound of weight lost. Also drink 16 ounces of Gatorade or eat one fruit.

Dinner (7 P.M.)

2 oz. grilled teriyaki chicken	2 proteins
1 cup wild rice	2 grains
3 cups mixed greens and vegetables	3 vegetables
1 small whole wheat roll	1 grain
¼ avocado (if fat intake is low)	2 healthy fats
2 TB. lite Caesar dressing	2 healthy fats

For 2,400 calories, add the following:

>   3 grains
>
>   1 protein
>
>   0 fruit
>
>   1 dairy
>
>   0 vegetable
>
>   1 fat

For 2,700 calories, add the following:

>   6 grains
>
>   2 proteins
>
>   0 fruit
>
>   2 dairy
>
>   0 vegetables
>
>   2 fat

For 3,000 calories, add the following:

>   9 grains
>
>   3 proteins
>
>   0 fruits
>
>   3 milk
>
>   0 vegetables
>
>   0–3 fats

Fueling Up Before, During, and After the Event

If you're a competitive athlete, the following information will help you to better plan your nutrient intake when you're competing. The food you eat every day builds a solid foundation for your efforts. What you eat before, during, and after your event is like the icing on the cake.

Pre-Event Fueling

The rule of thumb with pre-event/workout timing is as follows:

3–4 hours before 700–800 calories

2–3 hours before 500–600 calories

1–2 hours before 200–400 calories

>1 hour before 50–200 calories

3–4 hours before

2 grains

1 fat

3 fruits or 12 oz. sports drink and 1 fruit

English muffin	2 grains
1½ tsp. natural peanut butter	1 fat
12 oz. sports drink, ½ banana	(equivalent of 3 fruits)

2–3 hours before

1½ grains

3 fruits

1 dairy

1 fat

3 oz. whole-wheat bagel	1½ grain
3 cups mixed fresh fruit	3 fruits
fat-free yogurt	1 dairy
6 roasted almonds	1 fat

1–2 hours before

3 vegetables

1 fruit

2 grains

3 cups mixed raw vegetables	3 vegetables
1 peach	1 fruit
2 oz. fat-free crackers	2 grains

>1 hour before

1½ grain	
1 fruit	
1½ oz. bagel chips	1½ grain
1 pear	1 fruit

During-the-Event Fueling

If your activity lasts longer than 90 minutes and is continuous, eating 30 to 60 grams of carbohydrates every hour will help maintain your blood glucose levels. Dietary carbohydrates supply glucose to the muscles when stored carbohydrates are low.

Good sources of carbohydrates for during-the-event fueling include the following:

◆ Sports bars

◆ Sports drinks—16 to 20 ounces

◆ Grain products, such as whole-wheat or plain mini bagels (2 to 4 ounces)

◆ Liquid meals

◆ Fruits, such as a ripe banana, raisins, etc.

◆ Sports gels made from brown-rice syrup or maltodextrins

Experiment with these before you compete—during a practice session is a good time. Trying new things the day of competition is never a good idea. If what you eat doesn't agree with you, all of your hard work is for nothing.

Post-Event Fueling

Following a good post-event eating program is one of the two best ways to improve your workouts and performance (the other is making sure you're adequately hydrated at all times). As you may recall from Chapter 2, your body uses glucose at all times, not just when you're being active. For this reason, it is extremely important to replenish your glycogen stores after you compete. If you don't get them back to where they were before your event, you run the risk of being a little low on glycogen the next time you work out. If you continue along these lines, your workouts will get harder and harder as you remain a little low on fuel.

There is a narrow window of time—about two hours after a workout or competition—during which you can maximize glucose uptake. For optimal levels, do the following:

◆ If you're training hard, you need to eat at least 1 to 1.5 grams of carbohydrates per kilogram of body weight (2.2 pounds) within 30 minutes after your workout or event, and an additional 1 to 1.5 grams of carbs per kg within two hours after your workout.

◆ For medium training, eat 0.5 to 0.75 grams of carbohydrates per kg of body weight within 30 minutes.

Hydration for Performance

To achieve peak performance, the goal is to consistently replace any fluids you are likely to lose during your workout or event.

The following is a formula for determining a "serious" athlete's optimal fluid needs:

◆ Two to three hours before a workout or competition, drink 2 cups (16 oz.) of fluids.

◆ One hour before a workout or competition, drink 1 cup (8 oz.) of fluids.

◆ Fifteen minutes before the event or workout, drink ¹/₂ cup (4 oz.) of fluid.

◆ Immediately before the workout or competition, weigh and record your weight.

◆ Every 10 to 20 minutes during the workout or competition, drink ¹/₂ cup of fluid.

◆ Right after a workout or competition, weigh yourself. Drink 3 cups (24 oz.) of fluid for every pound of weight lost.

Fluid Replacement Chart

Weight Loss (lb)	Ounces	Cups
¹/₄	6	³/₄
¹/₂	12	1¹/₂
³/₄	18	2¹/₄
1	24	3

continues

Fluid Replacement Chart   (continued)

Weight Loss (lb)	Ounces	Cups
$1^{1}/_{4}$	30	$3^{3}/_{4}$
$1^{1}/_{4}$	36	$4^{1}/_{2}$
$1^{3}/_{4}$	42	$5^{1}/_{4}$
2	48	6
$2^{1}/_{4}$	54	$6^{3}/_{4}$
$2^{1}/_{2}$	60	$7^{1}/_{2}$
$2^{3}/_{4}$	66	$8^{1}/_{4}$
3	72	9
$3^{1}/_{4}$	78	$9^{3}/_{4}$
$3^{1}/_{2}$	84	$10^{1}/_{2}$
$3^{3}/_{4}$	90	$11^{1}/_{4}$
4	96	12
$4^{1}/_{4}$	102	$12^{3}/_{4}$
$4^{1}/_{2}$	108	$13^{1}/_{2}$
$4^{3}/_{4}$	114	$14^{1}/_{4}$
5	120	15

You might need to make some additional adjustments when working out or playing in particularly hot weather. Use the chart here to help you keep track of everything.

Experiment with this formula and adjust accordingly for each athletic activity until your weight remains the same from the start of the activity through to the very end.

Fluid Record Chart

Event	Time	Weight Before	Weight After	Difference	Intensity of Activity	Duration of Activity	Weather Conditions (temp./humidity)

The Least You Need to Know

- The principles of sports nutrition bring out the athlete within and help all active people reach their goals, whatever they are.

- If you are exhausted after a meet or a practice, chances are it's the lack of fluid and nutrients that make you feel this way.

- Post-event fueling with carbohydrates is essential for replenishing the body's supply of glucose.

- To achieve peak performance, you need to consistently replace any fluids you are likely to lose during your workout or event.

Chapter 4

Getting Into the Habit

In This Chapter

- ◆ Making and breaking habits
- ◆ Keeping new habits going
- ◆ Making a habit of reading food labels
- ◆ Planning for success

Habits can be our best friends or our worst enemies. They are formed over time, and before you know it, they can be very hard to break.

Being able to create new habits and break old habits is key to getting the results you want through a sports nutrition program. In this chapter, you'll learn how to identify your negative habits and replace them with positive ones. You'll also be introduced to some important habits that will serve you well for life.

Habitual Habits

A habit can be defined as an action or behavioral pattern—good or bad—that is regular, repetitive, and often unconscious. They start as early as infancy, and begin with observation. The brain processes information from the sensory nerves—our sense of taste, touch, scent, and hearing. Information then travels from the brain to the motor nerves to create actions. As we repeat these actions, our bodies eventually bypass the brain and subconsciously act without our even thinking about it. When this happens, you've gotten into a habit.

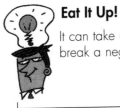

Eat It Up!

It can take up to a year to break a negative habit.

Positive habits have a delayed sense of reward and happiness. Negative habits are usually externally focused and meet an instant gratification. You only have to do something 20 or 30 times to create a new habit, regardless of whether it's positive or negative.

Many adults don't get the proper amount of exercise. Some may exercise but not at the level they should. Or they may not be doing certain things that they need to do when they exercise, so they don't gain much from the experience. Others might exercise too much. All of these behaviors are examples of habits. In most cases, people who have formed the habit of not exercising run the risk of developing problems like cardiovascular disease. Still, they continue to put their health at risk because they've gotten into the bad habit of not exercising.

Replacing the Bad with the Good

Before we talk about the habits you need to get into to optimize your nutrition, let's look at how to break a habit. The most important thing is to take full responsibility for your actions. You can't blame anyone else for what you do or don't do. The only person who can change you is you. Try as you might, you can't change someone else. You can be a positive role model, but it's not your responsibility to change someone else's habits, only your own.

Dawn Says

Once you have developed a new, positive habit, don't go back to the environment that was a trigger for the old, negative habit. Some people believe that the people you hang out with can be an influence, good or bad. When I was young, I thought this was foolish, but I have to admit that if I hang around positive people who don't let obstacles stand in their way, their influence helps me excel. Negative people bring you down.

To break a habit, you need to replace it with a better habit. If you just focus on the habit you're trying to break, you'll end up thinking about it even more. By focusing on a new habit, you can leave the old habit behind and allow the new one to become automatic.

New habits are formed through practice and repetition. Here are some guidelines for replacing the bad with the good:

- Identify the bad habit. Try to see why this habit even exists in your life, and what makes it so bad. Once people realize that a habit is negatively affecting their lives, it can increase their desire for change.

- Identify the triggers for the habit. If you snack when you're bored, try to disrupt the pattern that leads you to this behavior. Instead of heading to the refrigerator, brush your teeth or take a walk. If you snack while watching television at night, try taking up a hobby that keeps your mind and hands busy. Or maybe you're in the habit of not taking your vitamin and mineral supplements on a regular basis. Triggers for behaviors like these can be more difficult to identify, but not impossible.

- List the advantages of changing the bad habit into a positive one. For example, if your goal is to watch your portion sizes, you might list such things as decreasing your body fat, moving with fewer aches and pains, doing more things with your kids or grandkids, being able to fit into the size-10 jeans that have been hanging in your closet for too long, and so on.

- Set a deadline for getting rid of your habit. Make it realistic and give yourself enough time to accomplish it. Set small goals rather than big ones. Don't try to do too much at once. For example, instead of saying, "Okay, now I'm going to drink 80 ounces of water a day," start out by drinking 8 ounces a day for five to seven days a week for two weeks, and build from there.

- Say no to excuses. Once you have set a starting time, stick to it. This will ensure that you begin working on your goal right away and it's not put off and forgotten.

- Visualize your success. Going back to the water example, see yourself drinking the water, enjoying the taste, providing your body with the nutrients it needs to perform at optimal levels, and drinking it every chance you get. Be positive and think in the present. Do some affirmations, such as, "I am energized and feel refreshed every day from providing my body with enough fluids."

- Last, share your goals only with the people who will support you in your new lifestyle. Surround yourself with the right environment to succeed.

Experimenting and finding out what methods work for you is one of the keys to success when exchanging old habits for new ones. You'll have to find out what works for you and what doesn't. For example, if you're trying to drink more water on a daily basis, you might have to get creative about working it into your routine. If you don't like carrying a water bottle with you wherever you go, you may have to make smaller bottles available everywhere you can think of—on your desk, in your car, in your tote bag, you name it.

Dawn Says

One of the biggest mistakes I see people make when they embark on a new habit is that they set themselves up for failure. Since they're looking for instant gratification, they launch into their new routine without planning ahead for it. They usually do okay for about a week or so. By the second week, they're falling off the wagon a little bit. By the third week, they're back to their old habits, or pretty close to it. You're always better off when you establish small goals that you can accomplish within a certain period of time, not immediately. The goal is delayed gratification, not instant gratification. It takes longer, but it lasts longer, too.

I also see people who lose weight but then gain it back within months. They forgot what their bad habits were, and those habits resurfaced when the goal was met. Nothing was replaced!

You might have to experiment with flavored waters or enhancing your water with fresh citrus slices if you're tempted to break your new habit because you're bored with the taste of water. It's important to keep going with your new routine until it becomes a habit. If you don't give yourself at least a fighting chance for success, or you dump your new habit because you slipped back into your old routine for a moment, you won't succeed. Being an "all or nothing" person only suppresses the old habit and doesn't allow the new one to form. Very few people are successful with this method.

Changing habits isn't always easy—in fact, it's usually darn tough. However, what you do today will affect your life tomorrow. Nothing will change unless you change it.

At this point, you might find it helpful to take some time to think about your nutritional and fitness goals and what you need to do to achieve them. As you do, think about the habits that you might have to eliminate or establish to help you meet your goals. Don't forget to give yourself credit for your good habits. You've earned it!

Now, let's take a look at some of the best habits you can get into when it comes to optimizing your nutrition.

Healthy Habit No. 1: Read Food Labels

Many shoppers just pluck the food off the shelves in the supermarket without thinking much about it. If you're one of them, this is a habit you're going to have to change. If you're going to be serious about eating right, you need to know what you're putting into your mouth.

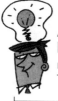

Eat It Up! _____

According to a survey of women shoppers, most of them don't read nutritional labels on a regular basis. Only 15 percent of those surveyed said they always read Nutrition Facts labels, and 61 percent said they sometimes read the labels. The remainder—23 percent—said they rarely or never read the labels.

This is a fairly easy habit to get into once you know how to decipher and interpret the information that's on packaged food. So let's get started.

Just about all packaged food comes with something called the Nutrition Facts panel printed somewhere on it that looks similar to the label here.

Nutrition Facts

Serving Size 1 cup (228g)
Serving Per Container 2

Amount Per Serving

Calories 250   Calories from Fat 110

	% Daily Value*
Total Fat 12g	**18%**
Saturated Fat 3g	**15%**
Cholesterol 30mg	**10%**
Sodium 470mg	**20%**
Total Carbohydrate 31g	**10%**
Dietary Fiber 0g	**0%**
Sugars 5g	
Protein 5g	
Vitamin A	4%
Vitamin C	2%
Calcium	20%
Iron	4%

* Percent Daily Values are based on a 2,000 calorie diet. Your Daily Values may be higher or lower depending on your calorie needs:

	Calories:	2,000	2,500
Total Fat	Less than	65g	80g
Sat Fat	Less than	20g	25g
Cholesterol	Less than	300mg	300mg
Sodium	Less than	2,400mg	2,400mg
Total Carbohydrate		300g	375g
Dietary Fiber		25g	30g

Sample Nutrition Facts label for macaroni and cheese.

(U.S. Food and Drug Administration)

This panel has two parts. The top part, or main section, contains information on serving size, calories, and nutrient information. This information is different on each food product. The bottom part, called the footnote, gives general dietary information about important nutrients. It only appears on larger packaging. The Nutrition Facts panel always takes the same format, regardless of the product. The only thing you might not see on every packaged product is the footnote.

All information on a Nutrition Facts panel is based on one serving, even if the package contains more than this.

Serving Size

Serving sizes are always stated in common-sense terms, such as pieces, slices, cups, and so on, followed by a metric measure—in this case, grams. The number of servings that the package contains is also noted.

Serving sizes are supposedly based on the amount of food that people actually eat, but in many cases these amounts either understate or overstate actual intake by quite a bit. If you're used to large portions, you might find that a package that is labeled as containing two portions might be plenty for just you. If this is the case, you'll be eating double the calories and other nutrient numbers stated on the package.

Calories and Calories from Fat

The next part of the Nutrition Facts label tells you what you need to know about the calories contained in each serving of the food product, and how many calories from fat they contain. In our example, there are 250 calories in a serving, with 110 of those calories coming from fat. To compute the percentage of fat in the product, just divide the calories from fat by the total calories. In this case, almost 50 percent is fat.

Nutrients

Next up is information on the specific nutrients contained in the food. All labels are required to list the following:

- Total Fat
- Saturated Fat
- Cholesterol

- ◆ Sodium

- ◆ Total Carbohydrate

- ◆ Dietary Fiber

- ◆ Protein

- ◆ Vitamin A

- ◆ Vitamin C

- ◆ Calcium

Eat It Up! _____

The daily value for protein is also listed if the food is meant for infants and children under four years old. If it isn't, none is needed.

Nutrients are listed as a percentage of daily value (%DV), based on a 2,000-calorie diet. By paying attention to these values, you can tell if the amounts of various nutrients in the product are low or high.

One thing you might notice is that there are no daily values listed for sugars or protein on this label. This is because there are no recommendations for the total amount of sugar to eat in a day. When it comes to protein, a daily value is listed only if the product makes a claim related to protein, such as saying "high in protein."

Nutrient Content Claims

Food manufacturers can also label their products as fat free, low in fat, low in sugar, and so on, based on the amount of these nutrients that the products contain. These claims are based on the same standardized serving sizes used to establish the nutritional information on the Nutrition Facts label.

Definitions of Nutrient Content Claims (Source: U.S. Food and Drug Administration)

Free — Synonyms for "Free": "Zero," "No," "Without," "Trivial Source of," "Dietarily Insignificant Source of." Definitions for "Free" for meals and main dishes are the stated values per labeled serving.

Low — Synonyms for "Low": "Little," ("Few" for Calories), "Contains a Small Amount of," "Low Source of."

Reduced/Less — Synonyms for "Reduced/Less": "Lower" ("Fewer" for Calories). "Modified" may be used in statement of identity. Definitions for meals and main dishes are the same as for individual foods on a per 100 g basis.

Comments — For "Free," "Very Low," or "Low," must indicate meets a definition if food without benefit of special processing, alteration; e.g., "broccoli, a fat-free food" or "celery, a low-calorie food."

Nutrient	Free	Low	Reduced/Less	Comments
Calories	Less than 5 cal per reference amount and per labeled serving	40 cal or less per reference amount (and per 50 g if reference amount is small) Meals and main dishes: 120 cal or less per 100 g	At least 25% fewer calories per reference amount than an appropriate reference food Reference food may not be "Low Calorie" Uses term "Fewer" rather than "Less"	"Light" or "Lite": if 50% or more of the calories are from fat, fat must be reduced by at least 50% per reference amount. If less than 50% of calories are from fat, fat must be reduced at least 50% or calories reduced at least ⅓ per reference amount.

Nutrient	Free	Low	Reduced/Less	Comments
				"Light" or "Lite" meal or main dish product meets definition for "Low Calorie" or "Low Fat" meal and is labeled to indicate which definition is met
				For dietary supplements: Calorie claims can only be made when the reference product is greater than 40 calories per serving
Total Fat	Less than 0.5 g per reference amount and per labeled serving (or for meals and main dishes, less than 0.5 g per labeled serving)	3 g or less per reference amount (and per 50 g if reference amount is small)	At least 25% less fat per reference amount than an appropriate reference food	"_% Fat Free": Okay if meets the requirements for "Low Fat"
	Not defined for meals or main dishes	Meals and main dishes: 3 g or less per 100 g and not more than 30% of calories from fat	Reference food may not be "Low Fat"	100% Fat Free: food must be "Fat Free"
				"Light"—see above
				For dietary supplements: calorie claims cannot be made for products that are 40 calories or less perserving

Nutrient	Free	Low	Reduced/Less	Comments
Saturated Fat	Less than 0.5 g saturated fat and less than 0.5 g trans fatty acids per reference amount and per labeled serving (or for meals and main dishes, less than 0.5 g trans fatty acids per labeled serving) No ingredient that is understood to contain saturated fat except as noted below (*)	1 g or less per reference amount and 15% or less of calories from saturated fat Meals and main dishes: 1 g or less per 100 g and less than 10% of calories from saturated fat	At least 25% less saturated fat per reference amount than an appropriate reference food Reference food may not be "Low Saturated Fat"	Next to all saturated fat claims, must declare the amount of cholesterol if 2 mg or more per reference amount; and the amount of total fat if more than 3 g per reference amount (or 0.5 g or more of total fat for "Saturated Fat Free") For dietary supplements: Saturated fat claims cannot be made for products that are 40 calories or less per serving
Cholesterol	Less than 2 mg per reference amount and per labeled serving (or for meals and main dishes, less than 2 mg per labeled serving) No ingredient that contains cholesterol except as noted below (*)	20 mg or less per reference amount (and per 50 g of food if reference amount is small) If qualifies by special processing and total fat exceeds 13 g per reference and labeled serving, the amount of cholesterol must be	At least 25% less cholesterol per reference amount than an appropriate reference food Reference food may not be "Low Cholesterol"	Cholesteral claims only allowed when food contains 2 g or less saturated fat per reference amount; or for meals and main dish products—per labeled serving size for "Free" claims or per 100 g for "Low" and "Reduced/Less" claims

Nutrient	Free	Low	Reduced/Less	Comments
	If less than 2 mg per reference amount by special processing and total fat exceeds 13 g per reference amount and labeled serving, the amount of cholesterol must be "Substantially Less" (25%) than in a reference food with significant market share (5% of market)	"Substantially Less" (25%) than in a reference food with significant market share (5%) of market Meals and main dishes: 20 mg or less per 100 g		Must declare the amount of total fat next to cholesterol claim when fat exceeds 13 g per reference amount and labeled serving (or per 50 g of food if reference amount is small), or when the fat exceeds 19.5 g per labeled serving for main dishes or or 26 g for meal products For dietary supplements: Cholesterol claims cannot be made for products that are 40 calories or less per serving
Sodium	Less than 5 mg per reference amount and per labeled serving (or for meals and main dishes, less than 5 mg per labeled serving	140 mg or less per reference amount (and per 50 g if reference amount is small) Meals and main dishes: 140 mg or less per 100 g	At least 25% less sodium per reference amount than an appropriate reference food Reference food may not be "Low Sodium"	"Light" (for sodium reduced products): if Food is "Low Calorie" and "Low Fat" and sodium is reduced by at least 50%

Nutrient	Free	Low	Reduced/Less	Comments
	No ingredient that is sodium chloride or generally understood to contain sodium to contain sodium except as noted below (*)			"Light in Sodium": if sodium is reduced by at least 50% per reference amount. Entire term "Light in Sodium" must be used in same type, size, color, and prominence. Light in Sodium for meals = "Low in Sodium"
				"Very Low Sodium": 35 mg or less per reference amount (and per 50 g if reference amount is small). For meals and main dishes: 35 mg or less per 100 g
				"Salt Free" must meet criterion for "Sodium Free"
				"No Salt Added" and "Un-salted" must conditions of use and must declare "This is Not a Sodium-Free Food" on information panel if food is not "Sodium Free"
				"Lightly Salted": 50% less sodium than normally added to reference food and if not "Low Sodium," so labeled on information panel

Nutrient	Free	Low	Reduced/Less	Comments
Sugars	"Sugar Free": Less than 0.5 g sugars per reference amount and per labeled serving (or for meals and main dishes, less than 0.5 g per labeled serving) No ingredient that is a sugar or generally understood to contain sugars except as noted below (*) Disclose calorie profile (e.g., "Low Calorie")	Not Defined. No basis for recommended intake	At least 25% less sugars per reference amount than an appropriate reference food May not use this claim on dietary supplements of vitamins and minerals	"No Added Sugars" and "Without Added Sugars" are allowed if no sugar or sugar-containing ingredient is added during processing. State if food is not "Low" or "Reduced Calorie" The terms "Unsweetened" and "No Added Sweeteners" remain as factual statements Claims about reducing dental caries are implied health claims Does not include sugar alcohols

*Notes: *Except if the ingredient listed in the ingredient statement has an asterisk that refers to footnote (e.g., "*adds a trivial amount of fat").*

"Reference Amount" = reference amount customarily consumed.

"Small Reference Amount" = reference amount of 30 g or less or 2 tablespoons or less (for dehydrated foods that are typically consumed when rehydrated with water or a diluent containing an insignificant amount, as defined in 21 CFR 101.9(f)(1), of all nutrients per reference amount, the per 50 g criterion refers to the prepared form of the food).

When levels exceed 13 g Fat, 4 g Saturated Fat, 60 mg Cholesterol, and 480 mg Sodium per reference amount, per labeled serving or, for foods with small reference amounts, per 50 g, a disclosure statement is required as part of claim (e.g., "See nutrition information for ___ content" with the blank filled in with nutrient(s) that exceed the prescribed levels).

Food Foul-Ups

Think those no-cal products you're using are really no-cal? Think again. Diet soft drinks do contain a small amount of calories. Spray-on oil or butter does, as well. One spray has less than 5 calories but if you pump that spray 10 times you've just added 50 calories to whatever you're making.

Here are some other nutrient content claim terms you need to know:

◆ "Provides," "Contains," or "Good Source." To use these terms, the food must contain 10 to 19 percent of the daily value per reference amount.

◆ "High," "Excellent Source," or "Rich In." The food must contain 20 percent or more of the daily value per reference amount.

◆ "More," "Added," "Enriched," or "Fortified." The food must contain 10 percent or more of the daily value for protein, vitamins, minerals, fiber, or potassium per reference amount when compared to the reference food.

◆ "Fiber." To make any fiber claim, the food must meet the criteria for either "good source" or "high." If the food is not low fat, the fat content per serving will also be listed.

◆ "Lean." To use this term for meat, seafood, poultry, or game, the product must contain less than 10 grams of fat, less than 4 grams of saturated fat, less than 95 milligrams per reference amount and 100 grams.

◆ "Extra Lean." Used to describe meat, seafood, poultry, and game. Food must contain less than 5 grams of fat, less than 2 grams of saturated fat, and less than 95 milligrams of cholesterol per reference amount and 100 grams.

◆ "Fresh." The food must be in its raw state and must not have been frozen or preserved.

◆ "Natural." While there is no set definition or regulation regarding the use of this word, using this word suggests that nothing artificial or synthetic has been included in the food that would not normally be in it.

◆ "Healthy." To use this term, the food must be low fat and low in saturated fat, contain 480 mg or less of sodium per serving, and provide at least 10 percent of the daily value per reference amount for protein, fiber, iron, calcium, and vitamin A or C. Seafood or game meats must have 5 grams or less of fat and 2 grams or less of saturated fat per reference amount and 100 grams, and 95 mg or less of cholesterol per 100 grams.

The FDA also allows food manufacturers to make certain health claims on their packaging based on the nutrients in selected foods and their relationship to certain diseases. For example, a manufacturer can say that a product is a "good source" of folate if the product contains at least 40 mg folate per serving. Thanks to a new FDA initiative, this information will soon be expanded to allow manufacturers to make even more health claims about their products. Labels will be able to tout the healthy benefits of such things as lycopene in tomatoes or omega-3 fatty acids in salmon as long as there is scientific evidence to prove it.

Healthy Habit No. 2: Keep a Food Record

As you read in Chapter 3, keeping a daily food record is a proven tool for helping people reach their nutritional goals. You can use the following chart as a basis for your record, or any other form that works for you.

When recording your foods, be as accurate and honest as you can. You only cheat yourself when you're not. Also:

- ◆ Record all snacks and "picking foods."
- ◆ Record all beverages, including water.
- ◆ Record any additional products you add to coffee or tea.
- ◆ Record any toppings or condiments.
- ◆ Record each food completely, such as fried chicken breast, broiled choice sirloin, etc.

Daily Food/Activity Record

Time	Food	Quantity	Hunger Level Before	After	Eating for Fuel or Habit?	Activity Type	Duration

continues

Daily Food/Activity Record (continued)

Time	Food	Quantity	Hunger Level Before	After	Eating for Fuel or Habit?	Activity Type	Duration

1 means you are starving

10 means you are stuffed

habit = feeling, thought, or mood

Keeping a food record can help you understand your eating patterns, which will help you when you move on to the next healthy habit—planning.

Healthy Habit No. 3: Planning

Planning your meals and your workouts is one of the fundamental elements of sports nutrition. Mapping out these activities will help you to attain your goals much faster and to be more aware of attaining them when you do.

Although this may seem impossible to do, you should put together a plan that covers at least two to three months—the time it takes to establish a new habit. Write down what you plan to eat and what you actually put in your month. Include activities and times.

More planning tips:

◆ Always be aware of your goals. Review these goals at least two times a day. This will help you remain focused and positive.

◆ Try to set only three goals a week. Many people overextend when it comes to goal setting, which sets them up for failure when they can't attain them all. Then they drift back to their old habits. Fast is temporary. Slow means a lifetime.

◆ Make it easy on yourself by planning out only as far as you find comfortable—a day, a couple of days, or a week at a time.

◆ Make sure you make plans for your plans. Don't forget to include things like trips to the supermarket. Plan the date and the time.

◆ Also make sure you plan for meals eaten away from home. How are you going to get your food to the workplace? What are your options if you eat out?

◆ Review your plan along with your goals.

◆ Make changes when necessary. Learn to go with change—that is life.

Eat It Up! _____

Have snacks on hand in your car or office in case of a change in schedule.

FOOD AND ACTIVITY PLANNER

What are my goal/goals for the week? (No more than three)

1. _____

2. _____

3. _____

Time	Food and Activity Planned	Time	Food and Activity Actually Eaten/Engaged In

What do I have to do to make this happen?

1. _____

   _____

2. _____

   _____

3. _____

   _____

4. _____

   _____

Remember, there is no short path to success. When you take a short cut, you usually have to go back and trace your steps. When you do the work on the front end by establishing good habits and setting goals and objectives, the chances of your having to start over from the beginning are much lower.

The Least You Need to Know

- Creating new habits and breaking old habits will help you get the results you want through a sports-nutrition program.

- Products labeled as having no calories do contain a small amount of calories.

- Keep a food record to help you understand what you eat, when you eat, and why you eat.

- When putting together your food and activity plan, try to create one that covers at least two to three months, which is the amount of time it takes to establish a new habit.

Part 2

Ready! Set! Eat Well!

Macronutrients, micronutrients, food pyramids, antioxidants—it's a veritable jungle out there when it comes to understanding the various elements of healthy eating. Combine them with what seems like a never-ending stream of nutritional research and reports that say one thing one week and another thing the next, and it's no wonder that most people feel like nutritional dunces.

If you're among them, it's time to go to school. In the pages ahead, we'll tell you what you need to know about the big guys—the macronutrient family of carbohydrates, fat, and protein, and why it's important to eat a healthy balance of all of them. You'll also learn about the micronutrients—vitamins and minerals—and the most important nutrient of them all—good old H_2O.

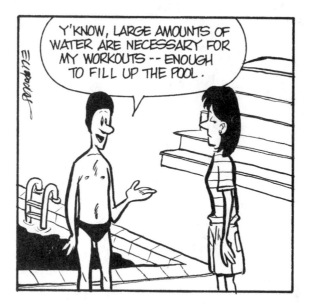

Triangular Truths

In This Chapter

- Getting to know the food pyramid
- Adapting the pyramid to your own needs
- Avoiding food pyramid pitfalls
- Another way to look at food groups

If you've spent any time at all looking into the basics of good nutrition (apart from this book, of course), you probably already know about something called the Food Guide Pyramid, or just the food pyramid. It may sound like a diet plan from ancient Egypt, but it's really a handy device for figuring out how to include all the various nutrients you need in your diet.

The food pyramid—called such because it's shaped like a triangle—has been around for the past decade or so. During that time, it has become the gold standard for nutritional planning. It's flexible enough to meet the nutritional needs for most people, and it's pretty easy to understand. It can also help you figure out what you should be eating every day. But it's not the only tool you can use.

All About the Pyramid

In a nutshell, the food pyramid is a device developed by the U.S. Department of Agriculture (USDA) to help people make food choices that will result in their eating nutritionally balanced diets. It's not meant to be a regimented food plan, but rather a general guide to good nutrition. It emphasizes eating a variety of foods from five main food groups:

- ◆ Group 1: Breads, cereal, rice, and pasta

- ◆ Group 2: Vegetables

- ◆ Group 3: Fruits

- ◆ Group 4: Milk, yogurt, and cheese

- ◆ Group 5: Meat, poultry, fish, dry beans, eggs, and nuts

The USDA Food Pyramid.

(USDA and DHHS)

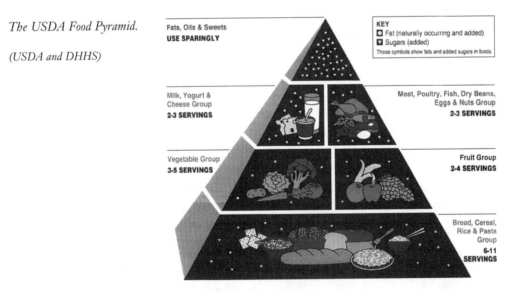

Because fats, oils, and sweets are also a part of our diet, the pyramid also includes them, but not as a recommended food group. These foods are to be "eaten sparingly."

Foods are grouped in categories based on their nutritional makeup:

Food Group	Major Contributions
Bread, cereal rice, and pasta	Carbohydrate, thiamin, riboflavin, iron, niacin, folate, magnesium, dietary fiber, zinc
Vegetable group	Carbohydrate, vitamin A, vitamin C, folate, magnesium, dietary fiber
Fruit group	Carbohydrate, vitamin C, dietary fiber
Milk group	Carbohydrate, calcium, riboflavin, protein, potassium, zinc, magnesium, vitamin A, vitamin B6
Meat and beans	Protein, niacin, iron, vitamin B6, zinc, group thiamin, vitamin B12, vitamin A
Fats, oils, sweets	Some fats and oils are good sources of omega-3 and vitamin E

The pyramid emphasizes grains, vegetables, and fruits as the major source of calories in the diet instead of foods that are high in animal protein and fat. Foods in the "no-no" category—fats, oils, and sweets—are at the top, indicating that we should limit our intake of them. From there, food is grouped by number of servings:

◆ Milk, yogurt, and cheese—two to three servings daily. Servings are 1 cup of yogurt or milk; 1½ ounces of natural cheese, such as Cheddar; and 2 ounces of processed cheese, such as American.

◆ Meat, poultry, fish, dry beans, eggs, and nuts—two to three servings daily. Servings are 2 to 3 ounces of cooked lean meat, poultry, or fish; ½ cup of cooked dry beans; 1 egg; 2 tablespoons of peanut butter or ⅓ cup nuts.

◆ Vegetables—three to five servings daily. Servings are 1 cup of raw leafy vegetables, 1 cup of other vegetables, cooked or raw; ¾ cup of vegetable juice.

◆ Fruits—two to four servings daily. Servings are 1 medium banana, orange, or pear; ½ cup of chopped, cooked, or canned fruit; or ¾ cup fruit juice.

Eat It Up!

The food pyramid was developed to accompany the U.S. Department of Agriculture's Dietary Guidelines for Americans released in 1992.

◆ Bread, cereal, rice, and pasta—6 to 11 servings daily. Servings are 1 slice of bread, 1 ounce (approximately ³/₄ cup) of ready-to-eat cereal, or ¹/₂ cup of cooked cereal, rice, or pasta.

By choosing the number of servings you eat in each category, you can control your calorie intake. The following chart will give you an idea of how many servings you can eat based on three different calorie levels.

Food Group	1,600 calories (most women, some older adults)	2,200 calories (most men, active women, teenage girls, children)	2,800 calories (active men, teenage boys)
Bread servings	6	9	11
Vegetable servings	3	4	5
Fruit servings	2	3	4
Milk servings	2–3	2–3	2–3
Meat servings	2	2–3	3

Note that there are no recommendations for the "other" group—the fats and sweets that are often little more than empty calories. There is a two-fold reason why there are no recommendations for food in this group. Sweets are just generally bad for you and have virtually no nutritional value. Added fats can be just as bad. The ones that aren't—foods that contain important omega-3 oils, for example—still must be eaten sparingly. If you're going to eat foods from this category, you'll need to decrease your servings in one of the more important food groups. Not a good idea!

Eat It Up!

There is room for some sweets and fats in a regular diet, but not much. If you're going to eat them, do so sparingly. It's okay to have a small doughnut once in a while, but eating a giant bear claw or caramel roll on a regular basis will put more of a dent into your nutritional plan than you'd like it to.

All in all, the food pyramid is a pretty good tool. It's definitely better than what it replaced—the "four food groups" plan (the milk group, the meat group, the bread group, and the vegetable and fruit group), which put too much emphasis on high-fat, high-protein meat and milk products as the key to good eating. Drawing from all the five food groups detailed on the food pyramid will definitely increase your chances of eating a balanced diet and getting all the nutrients you need.

This is a good first step along the road to good nutrition, and it might be an important one for you to make if your eating habits could use some improvement. But the food pyramid isn't Nirvana. The dietary guidelines it represents are pretty general, which means there is a lot of room for dietary sabotage. Here are just a few of the basic problems:

- Too many carbohydrate servings for most people. Add up the number of servings recommended in the three main carbohydrate categories—vegetables, fruits, and breads—and you end up with a diet that is way too heavy on the carbs.

- No distinction between whole grains and refined carbohydrates. There's a big difference in nutrition between a slice of white bread and a serving of brown rice, but the chart doesn't make this clear as it puts them both in the same nutritional category.

- Starchy vegetables, like white potatoes, peas, carrots, and corn, are lumped together with nonstarchy vegetables. Both are essential for a balanced diet. Again, however, there is a big difference in nutrition between the two.

- Not enough protein servings for certain people. Very active women and men, athletes (you!), people recovering from surgery or chemotherapy, and teenage boys need to eat more protein than the pyramid recommends.

- No distinction between animal proteins and nonanimal proteins. For nutritional variety and overall good health, many nutritionists feel that it's a good idea to eat at least one nonanimal protein daily.

- All oils are grouped together. While it's prudent to limit their intake, the pyramid makes no distinction between beneficial oils, such as omega-3 and mono-unsaturated oils, and saturated or hydrogenated fats.

Dawn Says

Order a spaghetti dinner while you're out on the town and you might be served two to three cups of pasta—four to six servings on the food pyramid. If your calorie requirements are such that you're eating on the low end of the recommended number of servings in the grains group, you've chowed down most or all of your daily allotment in one meal.

Another thing the basic pyramid doesn't do is go into detail on serving sizes. This information is available in the full nutritional guide issued by the USDA, but it doesn't appear on the pyramid itself. Because of this, a lot of people get into trouble when they use the food pyramid. They don't know what constitutes a serving size, so the serving sizes they eat run the gamut from about what the nutritional guide suggests to super size, and even super-super size. Not to pick too much on the grain group—this is where most of the problems reside—but very few people eat only a half-cup of pasta, which is one serving.

We'll discuss serving sizes in greater detail in future chapters. For now, just know that it's important to keep them under control or you'll end up taking in more calories than you should.

Making the Most of the Pyramid

As previously mentioned, the food pyramid is a pretty decent nutritional tool. However, randomly picking the foods you eat based on its recommendations won't deliver the best nutrition. Here's how you can make the most of the food pyramid by choosing the foods with the best nutritional content.

Food Group	Why Important	Best Choices
Bread, cereal rice, and pasta	Great source of B vitamins and fiber.	Products made with whole grains. Choose lower-fat foods.
Vegetables	Good source of vitamins A, C, folate, iron, magnesium, and fiber. Important for long-term health and fighting off illnesses.	All vegetables are good choices for different reasons. Eat raw or lightly cooked (steamed or sautéed in a small amount of oil) for best nutrition. Limit intake of fried vegetables.
Fruits	Good source of vitamins A, C, potassium, and fiber.	Always try to choose whole fruit over juice as much as possible.
Milk, yogurt, and cheese	Excellent sources of calcium, riboflavin, and vitamin D.	Choose low or nonfat products whenever possible.
Meat, poultry, dry beans, eggs, and nuts	A great source for B12, iron, and zinc.	Get good low-fat nutrition from this group by eating more vegetable-based protein (beans and tofu) and low-fat meats.
Fats, sugar, oils	Only about a teaspoon of fat is needed daily for the essential fats that our bodies can't make.	The feds advise to use products from this group sparingly, and with good reason. Not only do they add little to our nutritional well-being, but eating too much of foods in this group also means that you're missing out on the important nutrients found in the other groups.

The Food Pyramid for Athletes

As mentioned, the food pyramid doesn't meet the nutritional needs of certain populations, including athletes. Because people in this category are more physically active than the average population, they generally need to eat at the higher end of the scale when it comes to serving amounts to make sure they get enough calories to fuel their energy needs. Here's how to tweak the pyramid to meet your own needs:

- Milk group: Children under age 9 and active women and men should aim for three servings a day; older children, teens ages 9 to 18, and adults over 50 need four servings.

- Meat group: Two servings for children, teen girls, active women, and older adults; three servings for teen boys and active men.

- Vegetable group: Four servings for children, teen girls, and active women; five servings for teen boys and active men; three servings for older adults.

- Fruit group: Three servings for children, teen girls, and active women; four servings for teen boys and active men; two servings for older adults.

- Grain group: Nine servings for children, teen girls, and active women; eleven servings for teen boys and active men; six servings for older adults.

Even these recommendations might not cover your calorie needs, especially if you're working out at very high intensities. The serving recommendations here provide about 2,200 calories for children, teenage girls, and active women; 2,800 calories for teen boys and active men; and about 1,600 calories for older adults.

You can tell if you're eating enough if you are maintaining your weight during training. If you are losing weight, you might have to increase your calorie intake beyond what is listed here.

The Power-Fuel Chart

The food pyramid and the tweaks for athletes are good nutritional tools, but they're not the only way to look at the various food groups. The Power-Fuel Chart that follows is based on the one that accompanies the eating plans that Dawn personally develops for her sports nutrition clients, both amateurs and pros. It organizes foods based on protein, fat, and carbohydrate levels.

Dawn's Power-Fuel Chart

Food Group	Carbs	Fat	Protein
Fruits and Grains			
Fruit	15	0	0
Grains	15	0–2	3 (but not complete)

These foods mainly supply carbohydrates. They do differ in the nutrients they have.

Dairy and Meat			
Dairy	12	0–5	8 (complete source)
Meat	0	0–5	7 (complete source)

Dairy is high in carbohydrates but in the form of a disaccharide called lactose. This type of carbohydrate isn't absorbed very quickly. For this reason, dairy foods share similar characteristics to the meat group. They both supply similar amounts of fat and are a complete source of protein. They are similar in the macronutrients they supply, but differ in micronutrients—vitamins and minerals.

Vegetables			
Vegetables	5	0	2 (not a complete source)

Vegetables are also high in fiber, which slows down the absorption of carbohydrate into the blood stream. They're very important in the diet, but they can be considered neutral because they supply both carbs and protein and are low in calories—most of them, anyway. The only exceptions to this are the "starchy vegetables"—potatoes, corn, and so on. These are more like grains and should be considered in this category when it comes to the fuel chart.

Fats			
Fats Unsaturated, monounsaturated, polyunsaturated	0	5	0

The fats in this category are the "healthy fats." Your body metabolizes them differently, and studies indicate that this type of fat is good for your body—in moderation, that is. These fats can be found in oil dressings, nuts and seeds, wheat germ, flaxseed, avocados, and olives.

Saturated, trans-fatty acids, sweets and pastries	0	5	0

These foods need to be incorporated with care. They may taste great but they don't provide any healthy benefits or help your performance. In fact, they actually hinder performance and can damage your long-term health.

This chart works because athletes need to be more concerned about getting enough carbohydrates—and the right kind of carbohydrates—than any other type of food. This is why carbs are listed first for each food group. By knowing the number of carbs you need to eat to maintain your weight and energy level—we'll go into how this is factored in more detail later—you can pick the foods from the categories that will get you there. All you have to do is scan the chart to see which foods are the highest in carbohydrates. Then make your best picks based on fat content—staying at the low end of the scale on this, of course.

We'll get into more detail on using these tools in menu planning in chapters that deal specifically with the nutritional needs for various kinds of athletes. For now, keep in mind that serving sizes and nutrient balances vary from person to person. Regardless of what your personal requirements are, it's always important to choose foods from all the groups to meet your overall performance and health goals. Having a carb and a protein at each meal and almost every snack, combined with vegetables and a sprinkling of healthy fat, is one of the best ways to ensure that you're getting all the nutrients you need, regardless of your fitness goals.

The Least You Need to Know

- ♦ The food pyramid is a tool for eating a nutritionally balanced diet.

- ♦ You can control your calorie intake by choosing the number of servings you eat in each category on the food pyramid.

- ♦ Many people—athletes, teenagers, and older individuals—need to adjust the recommendations made by the food pyramid for their individual needs.

- ♦ To get the broadest range of nutrients in your diet, choose a variety of foods from the five food groups.

Conscious Carbohydrates: Part 1

In This Chapter

- ◆ What is a carb?
- ◆ Simple carbohydrates vs. complex carbohydrates
- ◆ Types of simple sugars
- ◆ How to recognize hidden sugars

When you exercise, your body uses the energy that is stored in your blood, liver, and muscles. That energy, as you already know, mostly comes from the carbohydrates that you eat. Carbs are crucial to your performance, but there is a big difference between the different kinds of carbohydrates and what they can do for you. Much as we might wish it were so, a soda won't provide the same energy and nutrients as a bowl of oatmeal.

In this chapter, we'll get to know carbohydrates in general a little better. We'll also focus on the first group of carbohydrates—the simple sugars.

Getting to Know Carbs

Carbohydrates are one of the three categories of macronutrients that our bodies need to function the way they should. Of the three macronutrients—fats and protein being the other two—they're the body's primary fuel source, which means they're the power behind your muscles.

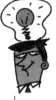

> **Eat It Up!**
>
> In the early nineteenth century, it was commonly believed that protein was the primary source of muscle power. This theory was based on the research and experiments of famed chemist Justus von Liebig, who was so widely revered that for a time no one dared dispute him. However, by the mid-1800s, several other scientists challenged von Liebig's beliefs, and proved that carbohydrates and fat, not protein, were what fueled muscular activity.

Like all organic compounds, carbohydrates contain carbon, hydrogen, and oxygen. They fall into two categories:

- Simple sugars, which, as you would expect, include sweet things like table sugar, honey, maple syrup, fruit sugars, and the like

- Complex carbohydrates, which come from plant sources and include grains, vegetables, legumes, beans, and seeds

What differentiates simple carbohydrates from their more complex relatives is their chemical composition. Simple sugars, as their name suggests, are relatively simple compounds. When several simple sugars link up, they become a complex carbohydrate.

All carbohydrates, regardless of whether they're simple or complex, are easily digested and broken down in the body, which is what makes them such a great energy source. They eventually turn into glucose and are stored in the muscle or liver. Your body can only store a limited amount of carbohydrates, though, so replacing them on a regular basis is key. How you replace them, however, can make a big difference in your performance. Even though the body converts all forms of carbohydrates into glucose, carbohydrates aren't equal when it comes to the nutrients and energy they provide.

How much carboyhydrate do you need to eat? Depending on how active you are, and your overall health goals, the amount varies anywhere from 45 to 75 percent of your total daily calories. In general, it's around 50 to 60 percent. For optimal sports performance, it's vital that you get at least 55 percent of your calories from carbohydrates. Eat less than this and you run the risk of glycogen depletion, which can severely affect your performance.

For the best nutritional benefits, be sure to select your carbohydrates from every food group that contains them—fruits, which are discussed in this chapter, as well as grains, vegetables, and dairy, which we'll discuss in Chapter 7.

Singing the Simple Sugar Blues

Simple sugars are a great energy source. Of all the carbohydrates, they get absorbed the fastest. That "bouncing off the walls" feeling you get when you eat a lot of candy or slug down a sugar-based soft drink is the direct result of the sugar these foods contain. But here's the bad news: You may feel an increase in energy, but the energy burst you get is only temporary. Because your body absorbs simple sugars quickly, they also leave your system faster.

We're programmed from the get-go to like sugary things—milk contains simple sugars—so we develop our sweet tooth pretty young. Eating a diet that's high in sugar, however, can be a precursor to many health-related problems, including periodontal disease, hypoglycemia, and diabetes. It can weaken your immune system and make you vulnerable to a whole host of problems beyond these, including yeast infections, a weakened immune system, osteoporosis, Plycystic Ovary Syndrome (PCOS), and adult acne, just to name a few.

Simple sugars also have almost no redeeming value when it comes to nutrition. They're little more than empty calories. But simple sugars aren't all created alike. To understand why some simple sugars are healthy and others are not, it's helpful to know a little more about how they're put together.

Simple sugars come in two forms:

♦ Monosaccharides, which are composed of just one sugar molecule. Glucose and fructose, the simple sugars found in fruits, honey, and processed foods, are monosaccharides. So is galactose, a simple sugar found in milk.

Eat It Up!

The typical American consumes an average of 135 pounds of refined sugar annually, which equates to a whopping 600 calories a day. That's substantially up from the turn of the twentieth century, when the annual per person consumption of sugar was 65 pounds.

Eat It Up!

According to a study by the USDA, people who eat large amounts of added sugars get less calcium, fiber, folate, vitamins A, C, and E, zinc, magnesium, iron, and other nutrients than people whose diets contain less added sugar.

◆ Disaccharides, which are formed when two simple sugars chemically attach to each other. A glucose molecule attached to a fructose molecule makes sucrose, otherwise known as table sugar. Glucose and galactose together make lactose, another simple sugar in milk. Maltose is formed by two glucose units.

Simple sugars are further categorized as natural sugars and refined sugars. Natural sugar is what we get from fruits and honey. Refined sugars are processed. The term includes not only the sugar listed in ingredient listings, but also brown sugar, glucose, fructose, and dextrose.

Fructose—the simple sugar that's contained in fruits and fruit juices—is absorbed very slowly by the body. Fruit is also high in fiber, vitamins A and C, and potassium. They also have a high water content and are low in calories. In other words, they give you great nutrients, more constant energy, and they fill you up.

Dawn Says

Need a quick pick-me-up after a tough workout? A 6-ounce glass of juice provides the daily requirement of vitamin C (60 milligrams) plus all the potassium you might have lost in an hour's workout, plus folic acid, a B vitamin needed for building protein and red blood cells. Orange, grapefruit, and tangerine juice have the most nutritional value. Other top picks are cranberry, apple, grape, and pineapple. Be sure to buy fruit juices that contain 100 percent juice and 100 percent vitamin C.

Top Fruit Choices

Fresh, Frozen, and Unsweetened Canned	Serving Size
Apple (raw, 2" across)	1
Applesauce	$1/2$ cup
Apricots (medium, raw)	4
Apricots (canned)	$1/2$ cup or 4 halves
Banana (9" long)	$1/2$
Blackberries (raw)	$1/2$ cup
Blueberries (raw)	$1/2$ cup
Cantaloupe (5" across)	$1/3$ melon or 1 cup cubes
Cherries (large, raw)	12
Cherries (canned)	$1/2$ cup

Fresh, Frozen, and Unsweetened Canned	Serving Size
Figs (raw, 2" across)	2
Fruit cocktail (canned)	$1/2$ cup
Grapefruit (segments)	$1/2$
Grapes (small)	15
Guava	1
Honeydew melon (medium)	$1/8$ melon or 1 cup cubes
Kiwi fruit (large)	1
Mandarin oranges (canned)	$1/2$ cup
Mango (small)	1
Nectarine ($1^1/_2$" across)	1
Orange ($2^1/_2$" across)	1
Papaya	1 cup
Peach ($2^1/_2$" across)	1
Peaches (canned)	$1/2$ cup or 2 halves
Persimmon (medium, native)	2
Pineapple (raw)	$1/2$ cup
Pineapple (canned)	$1/3$ cup
Plum (raw, 2" across)	2
Pomegranate	1/2
Raspberries (raw)	1 cup
Strawberries (raw, whole)	$1^1/_2$ cup
Tangerine ($2^1/_2$" across)	2
Watermelon (cubes)	$1^1/_2$ cups
Dried Fruit	
Apples	4 rings
Apricots	7 halves
Berries (mixed)	$1/3$ cup
Cranberries	$1/3$ cup
Dates	$2^1/_2$ medium
Figs	$1^1/_2$
Dried Plums (Prunes)	3 medium
Raisins	2 tablespoons

continues

Top Fruit Choices   (continued)

Fruit Juice	
Apple	¹/₂ cup
Cranberry cocktail	¹/₃ cup
Grapefruit	¹/₂ cup
Grape	¹/₃ cup
Orange	¹/₂ cup
Pineapple	¹/₂ cup
Dried Plum (Prune)	¹/₃ cup
V8 Splash (assorted flavors)	¹/₂ cup

Fructose can also be made from corn starch. This manufactured fructose is widely used as a food additive because it is almost twice as sweet as sugar and doesn't cost nearly as much. Because of this, you'll see it on many food labels as an added sugar. It's important to understand, however, that this doesn't mean that eating fruit is bad for you. What it does mean is that too much sugar in any form can be bad for your health.

Hidden Sugars

Even if you stay away from sweets or you read food labels carefully, you still can be consuming a large amount of refined sugar without knowing it. Nutritional labels do tally the sugar that occurs naturally in a product, but they don't have to list any sugars that might be added. Because of this, a food product that naturally contains sugar may also contain other types of sugar, such as honey, carob, corn syrup, and fructose, plus a host of other sweetening products that you may not recognize as sugar. This can be confusing and misleading.

Food Foul-Ups

Even foods that appear to be healthy when you look at the nutrition label might not seem as great when you scan the ingredient list. Unfortunately, if added sugars appear on the list, there is currently no way to know exactly how much has been added. Your only clue is ingredient order as they're sorted by amount. If sugars are fairly high on the list, they also factor heavily in the food product.

Breads, soups, cereals, cured meats, hot dogs, lunch meat, salad dressings, spaghetti sauce, crackers, mayonnaise, peanut butter, pickles, frozen pizza, canned fruits and vegetables, tomato juice, and ketchup are just some examples of where hidden sugars can be found.

To determine whether sugar is natural or added, read the ingredient list. You know sugar is added if any of the following products appear:

♦ Sucrose. We know it as granulated sugar or white sugar. Other products in the sucrose family include turbinado sugar, brown sugar, maple syrup, and molasses.

♦ Corn syrup. The most popular form of refined fructose. Food manufacturers like it because it is sweeter—70 percent sweeter, in fact—and cheaper than refined sucrose.

♦ Glucose. Also known as dextrose. Found in fruit, honey, carob, and corn. It can also be in refined form. It is about two thirds as sweet as sucrose.

♦ Sugar alcohols. Sugar alcohols, or polyols, add bulk and texture to food such as chewing gum and hard candies. These sweeteners are metabolized more slowly than sucrose and can be used in place of sugar by diabetics or those following low-carbohydrate diets. They're not completely absorbed by the intestine, however, and can have a laxative effect if too much is used. There are a number of different sugar alcohols. Mannitol, sorbitol, maltitol, and xylitol occur naturally in fruits.

Other sweeteners that also might appear on ingredient lists include fructose, brown sugar, honey, molasses, fruit-juice concentrate, maltose, maltodextrin, lactose, and galactose.

There have been calls for nutrition labels to contain more detailed information on sugars, including a declaration of added sugars in grams per serving and a corresponding daily value, and this information might get added in the future. For now, however, the only way you can tell if a product has added sugars is by reading the ingredient list.

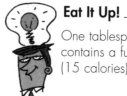

Eat It Up!

One tablespoon of ketchup contains a full teaspoon (15 calories) of sugar.

Healthier Sugar Choices

Given our genetic predisposition to enjoy sugar, we would be hard put to totally eliminate the sweet stuff from our diets. But it is possible to substitute products that have a little more to offer than just empty calories. While no sweetener can be considered a nutritional knockout, some are better choices than others when it comes to things like how they affect blood-sugar levels. Some also offer minerals and vitamins.

◆ Barley malt. This dark, sticky sweetener contains trace amounts of eight vitamins and several minerals. It has a strong flavor that may not appeal to some, but it goes well in hearty dishes. It's not as sweet as honey, but with its main ingredient being maltose, it enters the bloodstream slowly.

◆ Date sugar. Derived from ground-up, dehydrated dates, it's not a real sugar but can be used like it. Since dates are rich in fiber as well as a wide range of vitamins and minerals, date sugar contains some as well. It works best in baking, where it can be exchanged measure for measure for sugar. It doesn't work in beverages as it doesn't fully dissolve in water.

◆ Fruit-juice concentrates. These fructose-based products are made from the juices of various fruits that are reduced about one quarter through slow cooking. They're often used to sweeten and intensify the flavor of juice concentrate blends. White grape juice is a common fruit-juice concentrate. Be sure to choose those that haven't been stripped of their nutritional value during processing.

◆ Fructose. Also known as levulose, this simple sugar is derived from fruit sugar and closely resembles granulated white sugar. It's highly concentrated, so you can use far less of it to get the same level of sweetness as sugar—about half as much, in fact. It's believed that fructose doesn't have the same negative effects on blood-sugar levels as sucrose does.

◆ FruitSource. Made from a mixture of fruit and grains, it contains both simple and complex carbohydrates as well as small amounts of proteins, fats, vitamins, and minerals. It replaces both sugar and fat in baking, and can also be used in beverages and cooking.

◆ Granular fruit sweeteners. These products are derived from white grape juice and grain sweeteners that are dehydrated and ground into granules.

◆ Honey. There are definitely two sides to the story on this sweetener. It can rot teeth faster than sucrose (which it contains) and it can cause fluctuations in blood-sugar levels just like sucrose does. However, it also contains fructose, and the more fructose it contains, the less it affects blood-sugar levels. Because bees collect nectar from different sources, honey varies in levels of fructose and sucrose it contains. Clover honey, for example, is 60 percent sucrose, while orange blossom honey is 70 percent fructose.

Dawn Says
If you can, use only raw, unfiltered honey, which is minimally processed and contains all of its natural enzymes, proteins, vitamins, and minerals. The best sources are the producers themselves, who often sell at farmer's markets or roadside stands. The cloudier the honey is, the better. Unfiltered honey contains small amounts of bee pollen, which some studies suggest can help control allergies and hay fever symptoms.

- Maltose. Made from sprouted grains and cooked rice, which are mixed with natural enzymes and heated until the starch they contain turns into sugar. Maltose is about one third as sweet as sucrose. Barley malt and brown-rice syrup are two natural sweeteners that contain maltose.

- Maple syrup. The boiled-down sap of maple trees contains twice as much calcium as milk. Some syrups also contain traces of formaldehyde, so choose organic maple syrup if possible.

- Rice syrup. This traditional Asian sweetener has the mildest flavor of the liquid sweeteners and also contains trace amounts of B vitamins and minerals. It can be used instead of honey in cooking and baking as well as to sweeten beverages and cereals.

- Sorghum syrup. This old-fashioned sweetener comes from the sorghum cane.

- Stevia. Derived from a South American shrub, this herb can give foods a sweet taste. However, it can't be sold as a sweetener because the FDA considers it an unapproved food additive. Instead, it's sold as a dietary supplement. It's available in liquid, powder, and dried form.

- Sucanat. This product is made from evaporated sugarcane juice. It's then turned into light-brown granules that look similar to table sugar but are a bit larger. Because it comes from sugarcane, it contains vitamins, minerals, and trace elements. Sucanat has a distinct flavor, similar to molasses, that can take some getting used to. It can be used as an equal replacement for sugar in baking, cooking, and hot or cold drinks.

- Unsulfured blackstrap molasses. There are several different types of molasses; unsulfered blackstrap molasses is what's left from cane syrup after the sugar crystals are removed from it. It contains high levels of three important minerals—calcium, iron, and potassium.

Alternative Sweeteners

Sugar substitutes are at least 30 times sweeter than sucrose, which means that it takes smaller amounts of them to sweeten things to our liking. The American Diabetes Association calls sugar substitutes "free foods" because they have essentially no calories and do not raise blood-sugar levels.

The Food and Drug Administration has approved four alternative sweeteners for use in the United States:

- Saccharin. Saccharin, which was discovered in 1879, is the oldest sugar substitute and is 300 times sweeter than sugar. It comes as a white powder for tabletop use, and is also used commercially to sweeten baked goods, beverages, and jams. Use too much of it and whatever you put it in will taste bitter. There has been some controversy over saccharin's safety over the years, but it remains on the FDA's generally-recognized-as-safe (GRAS) list.

- Aspartame. Marketed as Nutrasweet, Equal, and Spoonful, aspartame contains phenylalanine and aspartate—two naturally occurring amino acids, which are the building blocks of protein. It tastes similar to sucrose but is 180 times sweeter and has no aftertaste. A packet of this sweetener is equivalent in sweetness to two teaspoons of sugar. Unlike other alternative sweeteners, aspartame contains calories and the body uses it like it would any other protein. However, we're not talking about many calories here—only four per packet.

- Acesulfame potassium. Marketed under the brand name Sunette, this sweetener was approved by the FDA in 1988 for tabletop use. It is now approved for use in baked goods, frozen desserts, candies, and beverages. Acesulfame potassium is about 200 times sweeter than sugar and is often combined with other sweeteners. It has a long shelf life and holds up well to heat when used in cooking and baking.

- Sucralose. Marketed under the brand name Splenda, sucralose is the only alternative sweetener made from sugar and is the newest artificial sweetener to gain FDA approval for consumer use. It is 600 times sweeter than its parent product, but it adds no calories to foods, as it can't be digested. Like acesulfame potassium, sucralose has a good shelf life and holds up well to heat. The FDA approved it in 1998 as a tabletop sweetener and for use in baked goods, frozen dairy desserts, fruit juices, gelatins, nonalcoholic beverages, and chewing gum. In 1999, it gained additional approval as a general-purpose sweetener for all foods.

Two more sugar substitutes—alitame and cyclamate—are under FDA review. It's the second time around for cyclamate, which was banned in 1970 after it was found to be a possible cancer-causing agent when it was fed to rats. Subsequent research failed to substantiate this finding, so the FDA decided to take another look. Cyclamate is approved for use in 40 other countries, including Canada, where it is restricted to tabletop sweeteners and pharmaceuticals.

In July 2002, the FDA approved another artificial sweetener called Neotame, which is made by the same company that manufactures aspartame. Unlike aspartame, however, the company plans to market this sweetener primarily to the soft drink and food industries rather than directly to consumers.

> **Dawn Says**
>
> The jury is still out over whether artificial sweeteners are that good for you in the long run. Some studies suggest that people who use them to shave calories end up eating those calories somewhere else, or that using them may actually make you hungrier. If you're serious about having more control over your sweet tooth, it's probably best to avoid using them as much as possible.

Sweet Tips for Reducing Sugar Intake

Although there are no set dietary guidelines for how much added sugar you should eat, the USDA suggests limiting added sugars to 40 grams (10 teaspoons) for a 2,000-calorie diet. That's not very much—remember the amount of sugar in a tablespoon of ketchup?

The best way to reduce the amount of added sugar in your diet is to focus on foods that are naturally sweet. Here are some more sugar-busting techniques:

- ◆ Be label savvy. Read food labels thoroughly, and keep an eye out for added sugars.

- ◆ Cut back or eliminate soft drinks. According to the Center for Science in the Public Interest, soft drinks are the single biggest source of refined sugar in the American diet. The average 12-ounce can contains 40 grams of the sweet stuff. Drink water, seltzer, low-fat milk, or juices instead.

- ◆ Reduce the sugar added to baked goods by one fourth to one third the amount called for in a recipe. The decrease in volume usually won't affect how the recipe turns

Food Foul-Ups

The USDA's recommendations don't apply to natural sugars like the ones you get from eating fruit and drinking milk. Don't eliminate these positive nutritional sources from your diet.

out. It sometimes will, however, so it's a good idea to experiment with this before baking something that absolutely has to turn out right.

- ◆ Use sweet-tasting spices and herbs, such as cinnamon, nutmeg, cloves, ginger, and coriander, to enhance the flavor of foods.

- ◆ Use alternative sweeteners that are sweeter than table sugar when possible.

It can take some time to re-educate your palate to enjoy foods that are lower in refined sugar, but the payoffs for doing so are big. But be careful not to replace foods that are high in sugar with those that contain more fat and sodium. Don't trade one vice for another.

The Least You Need to Know

- ◆ Carbohydrates are the energy source your muscles turn to first.

- ◆ For optimal sports performance, try to get at least 55 percent of your daily calories from carbohydrates.

- ◆ Avoid energy spikes by limiting the amount of foods you eat that have sugar added to them.

- ◆ Sugar can masquerade under many different names in food labels. Always read carefully.

- ◆ Artificial sweeteners can be an effective sugar substitute. The best way to break your dependence on sugar, however, is to not use them.

Chapter 7

Conscious Carbohydrates: Part 2

In This Chapter

- ◆ The power of plant foods
- ◆ Making good complex carb choices
- ◆ Understanding glycemic levels
- ◆ Fiber facts

It's hard to imagine how just a simple difference in chemical structure can make such a big difference in the nutritional value of a macronutrient, but this is exactly the case with complex carbohydrates. Foods in this group—grains, vegetables, beans, and the like—also contain simple sugars. When it comes to complex carbohydrates, however, those simple sugars are linked together by the hundreds, and even the thousands, to create foods that are—you guessed it—more structurally complex than those made up of simple carbohydrates.

Just like simple sugars, the body breaks down complex carbohydrates into glucose, which is the form that all carbohydrates must be in before your body can use them as energy. But, unlike simple sugars, complex carbohydrates contain other elements that are good for you, such as vitamins, minerals, and fiber.

For all athletes—recreational to competitive—complex carbohydrates are the best choice for fueling optimum performance.

Nutritional Stars: Complex Carbohydrates

When compared to simple sugars, complex carbohydrates are the true nutritional stars. They burn more cleanly and provide better and more direct fuel than simple carbs do.

> **Dawn Says**
>
> Complex carbohydrates—whole grain breads, pasta, rice, vegetables, cereal, and legumes—should be the mainstay of your diet. Depending on your activity level, they should account for between 45 to 70 percent of your daily intake, which equates to between 3.0 to 4.5 grams of carbohydrates per pound of body weight.

Complex carbohydrates fall into three categories: breads and grains, vegetables, and dairy products. For a balanced diet, you should select a variety of foods from each category. And try to choose whole foods—whole grains, whole-grain breads—as well as vegetables that are minimally processed. They contain more of the healthy nutrients you're after. Depending on the food, you'll also get a good dose of dietary fiber (more about this later), which will help you eat less and feel fuller.

Choosing whole grains and minimally processed carbohydrates also regulates blood-sugar levels. We'll discuss this in greater detail later in this chapter.

Breads and Grains

Bread and grain products are the densest carbohydrates, containing roughly 15 grams a serving. Because serving sizes are small, it's possible to pack in a lot of carbs when you eat these foods.

Cereals and Grains	Serving Size
Bran cereals (concentrated)	$^1/_3$ cup
Bran cereals (flaked)	$^1/_2$ cup
Bulgar (cooked)	$^1/_2$ cup
Cooked cereals (oatmeal, grits)	$^1/_2$ cup
Cornmeal (dry)	$2^1/_2$ tablespoons

Cereals and Grains	Serving Size
Grape-nuts	3 tablespoons
Grits (cooked)	$1/2$ cup
Dry cereal (ready-to-eat, sweetened)	$1/2$ cup
Pasta (cooked)	$1/2$ cup
Puffed cereal	$1^1/2$ cups
Rice, white or brown (cooked)	$1/3$ cup
Shredded wheat	$1/2$ cup
Wheat germ	3 tablespoons
Bread	
Bagel	$1/2$
Breadsticks (crisp, 4'' × $1/2$'')	2
Croutons (low-fat)	1 cup
English muffin	$1/2$
Frankfurter or hamburger bun	$1/2$
Pita (6'' across)	$1/2$
Plain roll (small)	1
Raisin (unfrosted)	1 slice
Rye (pumpernickel)	1 slice
Tortilla (6'' across)	1
White (including Italian)	1 slice
Whole wheat	1 slice
Crackers/Snacks	
Biscuit ($2^1/2$'')	1
Chowmein noodles	$1/2$ cup
Corn bread (2'' cube)	1
Cracker (round butter type)	6
French-fried potatoes (2'' × $3^1/2$'')	10
Muffin (plain, small)	1
Pancake (4'' across)	2
Stuffing, bread (prepared)	$1/2$ cup

Milk Products

Milk products are lower on the carb scale at around 12 grams of carbohydrates per serving. Again, it's tough to depend on them for your carbohydrate requirements as their serving sizes are also pretty large. Many people can't digest lactose, the simple sugar that occurs in varying levels in milk products. If you're one of them, try lactose-free products. Some milk products may not affect you as significantly as others.

Milk products are also a good source of calcium.

Product	Serving Size
Skim milk	1 cup
1/2% milk	1 cup
1% milk	1 cup
Chocolate milk (low-fat)	1 cup
Dry nonfat milk	1 cup
Plain nonfat or low-fat yogurt	8 oz.
Yogurt, low-fat, fruit sugar sweet	1 cup
Soy milk	1 milk

Vegetables

Vegetables lag pretty far behind when it comes to carbs per serving—only 5 grams in most cases. But they're low in calories and high in nutritional value. They're the best sources of vitamins A, C, potassium, and fiber.

Eating a diet rich in vegetables reduces the risk of cancer, high-blood pressure, and constipation. It also improves healing, and aids in recovery after exercise. As shown in the following chart, vegetables are packed with a bunch of vital nutrients, including potassium, that are lost when exercising. Eating complex carbs on a regular basis can help you replenish your supplies of these nutrients.

Vegetable	Amount	Calories	A (IU)	C (mg)	Potassium (mg)
Asparagus (cooked)	1 cup	30	1,200	40	275
Beans, green (cooked)	1 cup	30	675	15	190
Beets (canned)	1/2 cup	25	4	3	150

Vegetable	Amount	Calories	A (IU)	C (mg)	Potassium (mg)
Broccoli (cooked)	²/₃ cup or 1 large stalk	25	2,500	90	270
Brussel sprouts (cooked)	6–8 med	35	520	85	275
Cabbage (cooked)	1 cup	35	200	50	230
Carrot (raw)	1 large	40	11,000	10	340
Cauliflower (cooked)	1 cup	25	70	65	235
Celery (raw)	1 stalk	10	120	5	170
Corn (frozen)	¹/₂ cup	90	240	5	195
Cucumber with peel	¹/₂ med	10	125	5	80
Kale (cooked)	1 cup	35	9,870	80	290
Lettuce, iceberg	1 wedge	15	330	5	175
Lettuce, Romaine leaves	4 large	20	1,900	20	265
Mushrooms	4 large	30	Trace	5	415
Onion (raw)	1 med	40	40	10	155
Pepper, green/ red shell (raw)	1 large	20	420	130	215
Potato	Med, boiled in skin	75	Trace	15	580
Spinach (cooked)	1 cup	40	14,600	50	580
Squash, summer (cooked)	1 cup	30	780	20	280
Squash, winter (baked)	1 cup	125	8,400	25	920
Tomato (raw)	1 med	35	1,350	35	365
Tomato sauce (canned)	¹/₂ cup	45	1,200	15	485

Best Complex Carb Choices

As previously mentioned, complex carbohydrates help maintain consistent blood-glucose levels. However, some complex carbs—ones that are said to have a low glycemic index (abbreviated GI)—are better choices than others.

What's a glycemic index? The term refers to a tool that measures how foods affect blood-glucose levels. As you'll recall, all carbohydrates convert into glucose, which then enters the bloodstream. Some carbohydrates convert fairly quickly. Others break down more slowly, and enter the bloodstream at a more leisurely pace.

Foodie

Carbohydrates that convert quickly into glucose are also called quick-release. Those that take their time are slow-release. Some carbohydrates are both.

The glycemic index ranks foods based on their actual effect on blood-sugar levels. It starts at 100—pure glucose—and ends at zero. Foods that break down the fastest—and therefore affect blood-glucose levels the fastest—are at the high end of the scale. Some are so high on the GI index that they even score higher than 100. GI ratings of greater than 70 are considered high; 55 or less is considered low. Here are just a few of the high-end chart busters:

Food	GI
Dates	103
Sticky rice	98
Baked potato	93
Corn flakes	92
Rice crackers	91
Wild rice	87
Pretzels	83
Bagel	72
Popcorn	72
Watermelon	72
Corn (fresh)	60

And here are some foods with more favorable GI values:

Food	GI
Brown rice	55
Oatmeal	55

Food	GI
Kidney beans (canned)	52
Butter	47
All Bran w/fiber	38
Apple	38
Pear (fresh)	38
Tomato juice	38
Whole milk	31
Apricots (dried)	30
Lentils	29
Prunes	29
Cherries	22
Grapefruit	25
Peanut butter	14
Yogurt (artificially sweetened)	14
Broccoli	10
Lettuce	10
Mushrooms	10
Hummus (chickpea spread)	6

Glycemic index is a fairly new way of assessing carbohydrates. It's received some bad press because people have misunderstood how to use it. There's some very complex chemistry behind the concept, but it basically boils down to this: Foods on the high end of the glycemic level—white sugar, processed grain products, and other carbohydrates that are high in simple sugars—send blood-glucose levels up, which means that the body has to release more insulin to bring them down. Rely too heavily on foods with high GI levels, and your body has to keep manufacturing more insulin. Researchers now believe that increased insulin levels encourage the body to store calories as fat. It also causes cells to become insulin resistant. The result: obesity and diabetes.

Eating slow-release, low-GI food, such as whole-wheat pasta, stone-ground whole-wheat bread, high-fiber fruits and vegetables, and foods that contain fat and protein puts lower and slower doses of glucose into your bloodstream and reduces the workload on your pancreas. It also keeps you from experiencing wild swings in your blood-sugar levels. Using the glycemic index can help you make wise food choices that can keep blood-sugar levels balanced and prevent insulin-related health problems.

However, some people have taken it to excess and eschew all foods on the high end of the scale. This is the thinking, in fact, that led to the "pasta makes you fat" mantra that a lot of folks started chanting a couple of years ago. There's some truth to that statement—eating too much of any food can cause calorie overload, and it's pretty easy to eat more servings of pasta than we should. And pasta made from white flour scores higher on the glycemic index (38) than whole-wheat pasta does (37). But it scores higher, as you see, just by one point. Not only this, the chemical structure of pasta is such that you can reduce its already low GI by cooking it al dente.

As we said, this is pretty complex stuff. There are lots of factors—including fiber and fat content—that also affect the glycemic indexes of foods. Just know that it's important to balance high- and low-GI foods in your diet. It's more than okay to eat a high-GI carb like a white-flour bagel (GI 72), especially if you eat a low-GI carb, like peanut butter (GI 14) at the same time. The combo produces a meal that's far from busting the top off the GI scale.

Figuring Out Fiber

Another benefit of eating more complex carbohydrates is taking in more fiber when you're chomping down on all that good-for-you food.

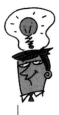

Eat It Up!

The fibrous part of carbohydrates contains the greatest concentrations of vitamins, minerals, and disease-fighting antioxidants.

The medical community has been pounding on us for years to increase our fiber consumption, and with good reason: Studies have linked high fiber intake with lower occurrences of some serious medical problems, including heart disease, diabetes, obesity, intestinal disorders, and hypertension; and several types of cancer, including colorectal cancer, prostate cancer, and breast cancer. Pretty amazing for a substance that has no nutritional value, isn't it?

Fiber Facts

Fiber is the exclusive substance of the plant world. It makes up the flesh of all nonanimal foods as well as their leaves, stems, roots, seeds, and coverings. There are various types of fiber in plants. Cellulose, the most abundant organic molecule on Earth, is primarily contained inside of plant-cell walls. Another common fiber called mucilage is found within plant cells.

The human body can't digest fiber, so what we take in passes right through us. However, while it makes its transit through our digestive systems, it works some miracles.

Soluble fiber, for example, literally clings to cholesterol and removes it from the body. Insoluble fiber moves waste through your intestines more quickly, lessening the chances of bad things remaining in your system too long. It also (we're going to get a little indelicate here) makes your bowel movements softer and more regular, which helps prevent constipation and reduce the chances of developing hemorrhoids.

Other side benefits of fiber:

♦ It slows down the rate at which carbohydrates are digested, resulting in slower and steadier glucose release.

♦ It contains micronutrients, particularly magnesium, which may help prevent diabetes.

♦ It expands in your stomach when you eat it, which helps you feel full longer.

The typical Western diet, with its emphasis on fiber-free animal foods and processed foods that often have most of their natural fiber removed, is amazingly low in fiber. In fact, the average American only eats roughly 12 to 15 grams of fiber a day, far below the 20 to 35 grams recommended in the FDA's dietary guidelines. In comparison, people living in Africa and India take in between 40 to 150 grams of fiber a day.

As mentioned, there are two different kinds of fiber—soluble and insoluble. Most foods contain both in various proportions.

Food Sources of Dietary Fiber

Food	Portion	Dietary Fiber (grams)	Soluble (grams)	Insoluble (grams)
Apple	1 medium	2.9	0.9	2.0
Orange	1 medium	2.0	1.3	0.7
Banana	1 medium	2.0	0.6	1.4
Broccoli	1 stalk	2.7	1.3	1.4
Carrot	1 large	2.9	1.3	1.6
Tomato	1 small	0.8	0.1	0.7
Potato	1 medium	1.8	1.0	0.8
Corn	2/3 cup	1.6	0.2	1.4
All-bran cereal	1/2 cup	9.0	1.4	7.6
Oat bran	1/2 cup	4.4	2.2	2.2
Cornflakes	1 cup	0.5	0	0.5

continues

Food Sources of Dietary Fiber   (continued)

Food	Portion	Dietary Fiber (grams)	Soluble (grams)	Insoluble (grams)
Rolled oats (cooked)	³/₄ cup	3.0	1.3	1.7
Whole-wheat bread	1 slice	1.4	0.3	1.1
White bread	1 slice	0.4	0.3	0.1
Macaroni	1 cup cooked	0.8	0.5	0.3
Green peas	²/₃ cup cooked	3.9	0.6	3.3
Kidney beans	¹/₂ cup cooked	6.5	1.6	4.9
Pinto beans	¹/₂ cup cooked	5.9	1.2	4.7
Lentils	²/₃ cup cooked	4.5	0.6	3.9

Source: Anderson, J.W., Bridges, S.R. "Dietary fiber content of selected foods." American Journal of Clinical Nutrition *1988; 47:440–7; and Bowes, A.D.* Bowes and Church's Food Values of Portions Commonly Used, *14th ed. New York: Harper & Row, 1985.*

Insoluble Fiber

Insoluble fiber doesn't dissolve in water and passes through your system largely intact. It's found in whole grains, wheat bran, nuts, seeds, and the stalks and peels of fruits and vegetables. Insoluble fiber aids your digestion. It increases stool bulk and speeds up its transit through the intestinal tract, which helps prevent constipation and irritable bowel syndrome. It also helps reduce the risk of developing hemorrhoids and diverticulosis.

Soluble Fiber

Soluble fiber dissolves in water and is broken down by the bacteria in your colon. It is found in a variety of foods, including oats, beans, peas, seeds, certain fruits and vegetables, and psyllium. Unlike insoluble fiber, soluble fiber forms a gel when it's mixed with fluids. Studies have shown that soluble fiber can reduce blood cholesterol levels, thereby lowering the risk of heart disease.

Increasing Fiber Consumption

The current recommendation is for 20 to 35 grams of fiber a day. However, some experts recommend levels as high as 60 grams a day. That may sound like a lot, but here's the good news: It's not all that tough to increase your fiber intake. It does, however, take paying closer attention to your food choices. The nutritional labels on packaged foods are now required to list fiber content, so it's pretty easy to make good choices if you read the labels as you shop. When it comes to nonpackaged items, just follow the FDA's recommended daily servings of fruit and vegetables (5 each) and servings of grain products (6 to 11). Doing so should get you "bulked up" in no time.

Instead of	Choose
White rice	Brown rice
White spaghetti	Whole-wheat spaghetti
Mashed potatoes	Baked potato with skin
Fruit drink	Fruit juice
Cooked carrots	Raw carrots

It's better to get your fiber from the food you eat instead of over-the-counter supplements. Doing so will also provide other important nutrients. However, you can also use a fiber supplement to help you reach these levels. Good ones have a 2:1 or 3:1 ratio of soluble to insoluble fiber for maximum health benefits. Supplements containing psyllium, derived from a plant native to India and Iran, are especially high in fiber.

Top-10 Food Sources of Fiber

Food	Fiber (grams)
Beans (legumes) cooked, 1 cup	12.0
Peas, green, cooked 1 cup	9.0
Raspberries, 1 cup	8.0
Bulgur, cooked, 1 cup	8.0
Rye wafers, 3 crackers	7.0
Wheat bran, 1/4 cup	6.0
Pasta, whole wheat, cooked, 1 cup	6.0
Oat bran, cooked, 1 cup	6.0
Squash, acorn, 4 oz.	5.0
Potato, baked with skin, 1 medium	5.0

When increasing fiber intake, do it slowly. It's definitely possible to overdo fiber. Taking in more than the recommended level can block the absorption of calcium, phosphorus, and other trace minerals, including iron. Excessive fiber intake also

> **Dawn Says**
>
> When you increase fiber in your diet, you must also increase water consumption. If you don't, you may end up constipated, because fiber needs water to expand in the gut and then move on through.

can cause bowel obstruction, which, if serious enough, can require surgery. Even in small amounts, increased fiber intake often causes gas and intestinal cramps. These common but temporary side effects usually resolve in a few weeks. If they bother you excessively, simply cut back your intake. There are also dietary supplements you can try—Beano is the best known—to help ease your way into a fiber-full life.

The Least You Need to Know

- ◆ Complex carbohydrates are the ideal fuel for athletic performance.

- ◆ To keep your blood-sugar levels at their best balance, focus on carbs that are minimally processed, such as whole grains, and whole fruits and vegetables.

- ◆ Foods that are high in fiber slow the rate of carbohydrate digestion.

- ◆ Eating foods that are low on the glycemic index, such as whole-wheat pasta, whole-wheat bread, and high-fiber fruits and vegetables, can keep you from experiencing wild swings in your blood-sugar levels.

Protein Power

In This Chapter

- Protein building blocks
- Animal vs. vegetable protein
- Complete vs. incomplete protein
- How to figure individual protein needs

The title of this chapter says it all: Protein is powerful! It's vital for tissue growth, repair, and maintenance—all important issues for athletes. But protein's power goes beyond this. It also plays a key role in your immune system, it helps make hormones and it carries nutrients throughout your body.

Protein has gotten a bit of a bad rap in recent years, thanks mostly to the debate over high-protein diets versus high-carbohydrate diets and concerns that eating too much protein can be bad for your health. Protein has its naysayers, that's for sure, but there's no denying the essential role it plays in keeping your body functioning like it should.

Steak and Eggs vs. Pasta and Potatoes

It wasn't too long ago that the common belief was that protein—and especially animal sources of protein—was essential for building strength and muscle. Since muscles are made mostly of protein, people thought that eating more protein would build more muscle. A typical training-table meal consisted of protein—lots of it—and not much else. Athletes chowed down on the classic protein combo—steak and eggs—in prodigious proportions. A lot was good and the more the better.

In recent years, nutritional research has shot down this theory. We now know that exercise, not extra protein, provides the building blocks for strength and muscle mass. Taking in more protein than your body needs will not build more muscle or build it faster. We also know that protein takes a back seat to carbohydrates for providing the energy needed for muscle-building exercise.

Not only this, but eating large amounts of animal protein—especially before competition—has actually been shown to hinder performance. Here's why: Animal protein is often laden with fat, and fat requires more oxygen than carbohydrates do in order to be metabolized. In other words, your body has to work harder to break it down. Neither proteins nor fat are converted to energy as efficiently as carbohydrates are. Plus, protein digestion generates certain byproducts that can adversely affect athletic performance. So, bye-bye, pregame steak!

> **Dawn Says**
>
> New research suggests that eating a small amount of protein—7 to 8 grams, about what you'd get in a cup of yogurt or skim milk—before strength training can be helpful for muscle development. Doing so makes the protein ready and available for muscle generation and repair after your workout.

As the focus shifted from high-protein/low-carbohydrate diets to high-carbohydrate/low-protein diets, many athletes either cut way back on their meat consumption or completely eliminated it from their diets. Pasta and potatoes, instead of steak and eggs, became the training table staple.

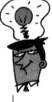

> **Eat It Up!**
>
> Protein makes up most of the weight of the human body that is not water—between 12 to 15 percent of body mass. The protein levels of different cells, however, vary considerably. Protein accounts for up to 20 percent of the total weight of red blood cells and muscle cells. Brain cells consist of only about 10 percent protein. Skeletal muscle contains the most protein and represents about 65 percent of the total protein in the body.

Now, before we go any further, know that there is nothing wrong with these foods. They are good sources of carbohydrates and they do contain some protein. They absolutely should be part of your diet, whether you avoid animal protein or not. However, pasta—and, for that matter, other grain-based foods—and potatoes aren't by themselves good replacements for animal protein. If you rely on them as such, you're opening yourself up for some potential nutritional problems.

In order for a high-carb diet to be nutritionally sound, meat protein has to be replaced with a healthy balance of plant protein from a variety of sources—beans, seeds, grains, vegetables, nuts, and so on. If this replacement isn't made, you won't get enough protein. Your body will take what it needs, mostly from your muscles, and you'll lose muscle mass. You also won't get enough of the nutrients that come along with protein, including iron, which is essential for carrying oxygen to working muscles, and zinc, which is necessary for healing.

To understand why this happens, you need to know a little more about what protein is all about.

Protein Profile

Like the other macronutrients—fats and carbohydrates—*protein* is composed of carbon, hydrogen, and oxygen. Unlike the others, protein has another ingredient—nitrogen. The addition of nitrogen is what makes protein unique in the macronutrient world. When nitrogen couples with the other elements, it makes amino acids.

All About Amino Acids

Amino acids are the building blocks of protein. There are 20 of them, and they are all different. Not only this, but they also can—and do—arrange themselves in a variety of different ways. As they do, they make different kinds of proteins.

Foodie _____

Protein comes from the Greek word *proteios*, meaning "of prime importance."

Eat It Up! _____

There are an almost infinite number of proteins that can be made through all the different ways that amino acids can link up. Linking together just 3 different amino acids can make 8,000 different proteins.

There are about 50,000 different protein-containing compounds in the body. Their chemical compositions and functions depend on how the amino acids are lined up. Here are some of the proteins that amino acids make:

- Hemoglobin
- Enzymes
- Antibodies
- Hormones
- Growth and maintenance proteins

Your body will also use protein as energy, although it doesn't like to. It will use it, however, if you don't take in enough energy from other macronutrients to keep the glycogen levels up in your muscles and your liver. This may not sound like too much of a problem, and it isn't if it doesn't happen very often, but the more that protein is taken away to create energy, the more it falls short on the rest of its functions.

Dawn Says

The one area in which protein is important for energy is for long-distance sports lasting longer than 60 to 90 minutes. At high intensities, your body will tap into something called branch chain amino acids (BCAAs) to perform. Leucine is a branch chain amino acid that the body uses up very quickly. It takes the byproducts of leucine and makes another branched chain amino acid called alanine. The liver then converts alanine into glucose—the main energy source we use when exercising. If we use it all up, we hit the wall.

Both people and plants make protein out of amino acids. Plants do it by combining simple sugars with nitrogen from the air and soil. Each plant makes proteins that are unique to it.

When you eat a food that contains protein, your body does the following:

1. Breaks down the amino acids that compose the protein
2. Combines them with the amino acids that it (your body) produces
3. Produces the new proteins that it needs for growth, repair, and other bodily functions.

Essential and Nonessential Aminos

Your body can make the majority of the amino acids it needs, but not all of them. Because of this, it's necessary to eat foods that contain the others. The 11 amino acids manufactured by the body are called "nonessential" because they don't have to come from outside sources. For humans, there are nine other "essential" amino acids that must be supplied by the diet. Your body can't store them like it does carbs and fat, so you have to eat foods that contain them on a regular basis.

Essential Amino Acids	Nonessential Amino Acids
Histidine	Glycine
Isoleucine	Glutamic acid
Leucine	Arginine
Lysine	Aspartic acid
Methionine	Proline
Phenylalanine	Alanine
Threonine	Serine
Tryptophan	Tyrosine
Valine	Cysteine
	Asparagine
	Glutamine

How does your body know how to assemble amino acids in the right order? Each cell in your body contains tiny protein factories, called ribosomes. They also contain DNA, which can be thought of as the instruction manual for making and maintaining an organism. The DNA coding in each cell tells the ribosomes how to assemble the amino acids for that particular cell.

When assembled, the amino acids form long chains, which then come together into coiled chains that take various shapes depending on what the protein's particular function in the body will be. There are two main categories of proteins—functional, which assist the chemical reactions in the body; and structural, which give tissues and organs their shape, structure, strength, and flexibility. Because animals both eat foods that contain amino acids, and manufacture their own, animal protein—meat, fish, poultry, milk, and eggs—is called complete protein, meaning that it contains the amino acids that your body needs. No one plant contains all the amino acids your body needs, which means they are incomplete proteins. Grains, for example, lack lysine but contain methionine. Legumes contain lysine and lack methionine. However, if you eat a wide variety of plant proteins, you'll take in all the amino acids you need.

One Protein + One Protein = Complete Protein

If you've dabbled at all with vegetarian eating, you may have heard about something called protein combining. What this refers to is eating plant-based proteins in combination to create a complete protein. Here are some examples:

◆ Rice and beans

◆ Peanut butter and whole-wheat bread

◆ Bean soup and a roll

◆ Pasta, vegetables, and tofu (such as manicotti stuffed with tofu and topped with tomato sauce and veggies, or lasagna made with tofu)

There are tons of other combinations you could make, but here's the good news: You don't have to make them at the same meal. Nutritionists once thought that incomplete proteins had to be eaten at the same time so that your body could derive the best benefit from them; however, recent nutritional research has disproved this. But, and let us repeat this again, you must eat a wide variety of plant proteins—the list below will help you choose them—to provide your body with the amino acids it requires to meet its protein needs. In other words, you can't survive on pasta and potatoes alone.

Vegetable Protein Sources

Food	Protein Grams
Almonds (1 oz.)	5
Black-eyed peas	7
Bread, whole-wheat (2 slices)	5
Broccoli	2
Butter beans	6
Cashews (1 oz.)	5
Chickpeas	10
Chili beans	7
Corn	2
Flaxseeds (1 oz.)	6
Garbanzo beans	7
Green beans	2
Green peas	4
Hummus (chickpea spread)	10

Food	Protein Grams
Kidney beans	8
Lentils	9
Lima beans	6
Navy beans	8
Oatmeal (1 cup)	6
Pasta (1 cup)	7
Peanuts (1 oz.)	8
Peanut butter (2 TB.)	8
Pinto beans	8
Potato, baked (small)	3
Rice, brown (1 cup)	5
Rice, white (1 cup)	3
Sesame seeds (1 oz.)	5
Soybeans	11
Soy burger	18
Soy hotdog	8
Soy milk (1 cup)	7
Soy sausages (one link)	4
Spinach	3
Spirulina powder (dried seaweed, 1 oz.)	16
Split peas	8
Squash	1
Sunflower seeds (1 oz.)	6
Tofu (6 oz.)	12
White beans	8

Note: All serving sizes are $^1/_2$ cup unless otherwise noted.

Note: The amount of protein per serving will vary depending on product. Always read labels for accuracy.

Dawn Says

Most plant sources of protein don't have a lot of fat, so you don't have to worry about it as much when you eat them. What you do want to do, though, is pick the plant sources that have the most protein—tofu, soybeans, legumes, beans, and so on—so you don't have to eat tons of them to meet your nutritional requirements.

Best Animal-Protein Sources

If you like to eat animal protein, we've got some good news for you: Not all of it is bad for you. If you stick to the protein sources listed here, you'll get all the good things that protein has going for it without high fat levels.

Animal Protein Sources

Food	Protein Grams
Bacon (1 slice)	5–8
Beef, lean, (USDA good or choice quality), including sirloin, round, flank steak	21
Beef, hamburger (cooked)	14
Buffalo	21
Canadian bacon	21
Cheese, low-cal (1 oz., 55 calories per ounce)	7
Chicken breast (without skin)	26
Cottage cheese, fat-free (1 cup)	30
Crab	13
Egg (1)	6
Egg white (1)	4
Ham (canned, lean)	18
Herring (uncreamed or smoked)	20
Luncheon meat, 95% fat-free (1 oz.)	5
Milk, skim (1 cup)	8
Pork tenderloin	24
Protein powder	16 to 30, depending on product
Protein bars	8 to 32, depending on product
Sardines (canned)	21
Salmon	18
Scallops	14
Shrimp	17
Swordfish	17
Tuna, white (canned in water)	25

Food	Protein Grams
Turkey breast (without skin)	26
Venison	13
Yogurt, fat-free or low-fat (1 cup)	10

Note: All serving sizes are 3 ounces unless otherwise indicated.

Note: The amount of protein per serving will vary depending on product. Always read labels for accuracy.

Protein Requirements for Athletes

Active people both burn more calories and need more calories to keep them going. They also need more protein than sedentary people do, but not by much. As mentioned in Chapter 2, the recommended daily amount of protein is 0.8 gram per kg of body weight, or about 0.4 to 0.45 per pound. If you are active, your protein requirements will range anywhere from 0.55 to 0.8 grams per pound. People who compete in endurance sports/long-distance sports should eat around 0.8 grams per pound; bodybuilders should be around 0.7 to 0.9 grams. If you're trying to lose weight, you should eat around 0.7 to 1.0 grams. Teenage athletes generally need around 0.9 to 1.0 grams per pound.

Because protein needs can vary quite a bit, there really isn't one exact figure to go by when determining your protein needs. To get an idea of what could be a healthy range for you, simply multiply your body weight by the number of grams in the category you fit into. For example, if you weigh 150 pounds and you're working out regularly at a fairly decent intensity level, you would need anywhere from 82.5 to 120 grams of protein per day to keep you going.

Food Foul-Ups

It is not necessary to take protein supplements to meet your protein needs, regardless of what all those fancy ads that promote these products say. You can easily get all the protein you need by eating real foods, not by drinking protein shakes and eating protein bars. Taking supplemental amino acids is another nice way to line the pockets of the companies that manufacture them. There is no evidence supporting their ability to increase muscle mass or improve muscular strength, power, or endurance.

If you take a look at the charts in this chapter, you can see how quickly you can meet your protein needs if you're eating animal proteins. For example, 3 ounces of chicken breast—one serving—has 26 grams of protein. Now, 3 ounces of chicken really isn't that much—it's about the size of a small clenched fist—and most people eat at least double this—6 ounces—in one serving. If you're one of them, you're already up to 52 grams of protein for the day. If you're eating at the low end of the scale for a 150-pound person, you've already taken in more than 50 percent of your daily protein needs—and that's just at one meal.

This is why it is so easy to overdo protein when you're relying on animal sources. Switch to plant proteins, and you'll be able to eat a lot more food and not go overboard on the amount of protein you take in at the same time.

The Dangers of Too Much Protein

Is there a clear and present danger if you eat too much protein? To a certain extent, yes. Your body knows its protein requirements, and it will only use as much as it needs. What protein you eat that you don't use might go to energy, but it usually is just extra calories, and they have to go somewhere. That somewhere usually ends up as extra pounds. Plus, if you're eating animal protein, it's accompanied by fat, which is another contributor to excess weight and other health concerns.

The other reason why high-protein diets can be unhealthy is that they can overburden your kidneys. When protein is metabolized, it leaves behind ammonia as a waste product. Ammonia is highly toxic to the body—among other things, it can cause liver and kidney damage and failure. To protect itself, the body converts it to urea, which is less toxic but is still something your body needs to get rid of in a hurry. The kidneys filter urea from the blood and send it to the bladder in the urine. The more urea that your body creates, the harder the kidneys have to work to get rid of it.

> **Dawn Says**
>
> Wondering how much protein you should eat? Your best bet is to determine your needs based on the ranges in this chapter and look at all the different foods you can eat to stay in your particular range. If you're trying to decrease the amount of animal protein in your diet, keep your servings of it small, and accompany them with lots of vegetables and grains.

High-protein diets can result in quick weight loss, which makes them popular among athletes who need to drop a few pounds in a hurry. However, much of the weight lost on these diets, especially in the first few days, is water loss, as the kidneys need to take water out of your body to get rid of urea. And, although it may not seem like it, you usually take in fewer calories on these diets, which in itself will cause you to lose weight.

The other pitfalls of high-protein diets include these:

◆ Ketosis. Diets that are high in protein and fat don't contain enough carbohydrates, which are essential for efficient fat burning. When fats don't break down correctly, acid-like substances called ketone bodies develop. When they accumulate, they cause an increase in the acidity in the body's fluids called ketosis, or acidosis. Symptoms of ketosis include dizziness, nausea, fatigue, confusion, and abdominal pain. It will also make your breath smell bad—something like a cross between apples or pears and nail polish remover—as your lungs will exhale some of the ketones as gas.

◆ Osteoporosis. High-protein diets cause calcium loss as it is excreted, along with other important minerals, in the urine. Calcium can also build up in the kidneys, leading to kidney stones.

◆ Gout. Sometimes called "the disease of kings" because people who eat rich diets are more susceptible to it, gout is a painful arthritic-like condition caused by the accumulation of uric acid around joints, tendons, and other body tissues. It can also be caused by eating foods that are high in purines, such as certain meats and seafood, which metabolize to uric acid in the body. Some dried peas and beans are also high in it.

With protein, as with all the other macronutrients, the key is balance. Know what your protein needs are, make wise choices of the foods that provide it, and protein will be a powerful ally in your nutritional game plan.

The Least You Need to Know

◆ Protein is made from 20 different amino acids.

◆ The body can make most of the amino acids it needs. However, "essential amino acids," which the body can't make, must come from food.

◆ "Complete proteins" are animal proteins that contain all nine essential amino acids. Vegetable proteins are considered "incomplete proteins" because they don't have one or more of the essential amino acids or don't have enough of them.

◆ Eating more protein than your body will use can result in weight gain, increased lipid levels, and dehydration caused by increased urination.

◆ Athletes need more protein than people who aren't very active, but not that much more.

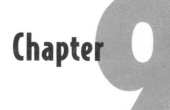
Fat and Fitness

In This Chapter

- The benefits of dietary fat
- Healthy vs. unhealthy fat
- Good vs. bad cholesterol
- Recommended fat-consumption levels

Fat is a big dietary bugaboo these days. We've heard so much about its evils that it's hard to believe there is anything good about it. But there is. Yes, eating too much fat—especially the wrong kinds of fat—can lead to lots of problems—obesity, heart disease, and cancer among them. However, fat is an important nutrient and eating too little of it can also create a laundry list of problems.

While just about everyone can afford to cut some fat out of his or her diet, including some fat in one's eating plan is a good thing. The goal is to strike a healthy level of fat intake, and to know which fats are okay to eat and which you should avoid, which is what this chapter is all about.

Facts on Fat

Fat is the most calorie dense of all the macronutrients, weighing in at 9 calories per gram. Because it's so calorie dense, it's an important fuel for athletes. The body can only store a limited amount of carbohydrate—about 2,000 calories. When those stores are depleted, we dip into our fat stores—about 40,000 calories, give or take—to keep us going. What's more, the better trained you are, the more efficiently you'll use and burn fat. In well-trained, well-nourished individuals, fat can provide as much as 80 to 90 percent of the body's energy needs. (Turn to Chapter 2 for more on how the body uses fat for fuel.)

Foodie

Fat-soluble vitamins are those that dissolve in fat.

Here are other reasons why dietary fat is important:

- It's essential for transporting the *fat-soluble* vitamins A, D, E, and K. Without fat to circulate, store, and absorb these vitamins, the body can't use them. It's like they're waiting at the bus stop, but the bus never comes.

- It protects the body's organs from injury. Approximately 4 percent of the fat stored in the body is used to cushion such vital organs as the heart, liver, kidneys, spleen, brain, and spinal cord.

- It protects the body from cold. Subcutaneous fat—the fat that's stored just under the skin—is necessary for weathering cold temperatures. On the other hand, too much body fat makes it more difficult to regulate body temperatures in hot weather as it literally prevents heat from escaping from the body.

- It supplies essential fatty acids like linoleic acid, gamma linolenic acid, and alpha linolenic acid, that the body can't manufacture.

But wait, there are even more good things about fat. It's vital for cell growth and support. Our skin and hair looks lustrous and healthy when we have adequate levels of fat in our systems, but dry and lifeless without it. Children who don't eat enough fat don't grow properly. Without fat, our metabolisms don't function as well as they should either.

To a certain extent, we're genetically programmed to like the taste of fat, which is a good thing since it's necessary to have a certain amount in our diets to stay healthy. Food that has some fat in it or added to it generally tastes better to us than food that doesn't, which is a big reason why downing a handful of french fries is often much more pleasurable than eating a baked potato with nothing on it. Eating a little fat also helps us feel fuller when we eat because it stays in our stomach longer than either carbohydrates or protein does.

Much of the flavor and aroma contained in foods and seasonings come alive when combined with fat. Chocolate-chip cookie dough doesn't smell like much when it's sitting in a bowl. Put it in a 350-degree oven, however, and it's a whole different story. It's not the flour and the eggs that smell so good. It's the butter and the chocolate (which contains cocoa fat) combined with those ingredients that set our salivary glands on high alert.

The good news is that fat, in and of itself, is not the villain in our diets. The problem lies more with the kinds of fats that are prevalent in the modern diet.

> **Food Foul-Ups** _____
>
> Significantly reducing fat intake below the recommended daily allowance can depress the body's level of the fat-soluble vitamins—A, D, E, and K—which can ultimately lead to vitamin deficiency.

Fat vs. Fat

Fats, or *lipids*, to call them by their more formal name, are not all created the same. While they share some basic traits, their chemical compositions are different and they affect the body in different ways. Some are definitely more harmful than others, which is why it's important to know the difference between them.

First, some basic fat chemistry. Like carbohydrates, lipids are composed of carbon, hydrogen, and oxygen atoms. However, lipid molecules differ significantly from carbohydrates in how their atoms are linked—unlike carbohydrate molecules, lipid molecules have a high radio of hydrogen to oxygen.

In the body, the majority of fat travels around in the form of fatty acids that hook up with a type of molecule called *glycerol*. Glycerol has three carbon atoms, which are what the fatty acids link to. When three fatty acids couple onto a carbon atom, they form a triglyceride. Triglycerides are the kind of fat we store in our fat cells and comprise most of the fat that circulates in our blood. They also are the main type of fat found in food, accounting for 98 percent of the fat we eat.

> **Foodie** _____
>
> **Lipids** are fats, oils, fatty acids, and compounds derived from them. **Glycerol,** a form of alcohol, is a simple compound of carbon, hydrogen, and oxygen that is produced when glucose is metabolized.

All fats and oils are primarily mixtures of different types of triglycerides. Depending on their chemical composition, triglycerides can be one of the following:

- Saturated, meaning that they carry as many hydrogen atoms as chemically possible. These fats are the most dangerous kind and are the leading contributor to high blood cholesterol and to heart disease. They are solid at room temperature and primarily come from animal sources.

- Monounsaturated. These fats contain one double-coupled carbon chain, which simply means that they're not completely saturated with hydrogen atoms. Studies have shown that monounsaturated fats can help lower blood cholesterol. They are liquid at room temperature and come from plant sources.

- Polyunsaturated. Fats in this category have two or more double carbon bonds, which means that they are even less saturated than monounsaturated fats. Fats in this category—especially those found in fish—have been proven to reduce the risk of heart disease. They, too, are liquid at room temperature.

Saturated Fats and Oils	Monounsaturated Oils	Polyunsaturated Oils
Animal fat	Almond oil	Corn oil
Butter fat	Canola oil	Cottonseed oil
Coconut oil	Olive oil	Fish oil
Palm kernel oil	Peanut oil	Flaxseed oil
Palm oil		Grapeseed oil
		Safflower oil
		Sesame oil
		Soybean oil
		Sunflower oil
		Walnut oil

Food Foul-Ups

Even though some fats are better for you than others, it doesn't mean you can eat them with abandon. Eating too much fat will make you fat—and at 9 calories per gram, those fat calories can add up in hurry.

All food that contains fat consists of both saturated and unsaturated fatty acids, mixed together in different proportions. Butter, for example, contains about 62 percent saturated fatty acids. Coconut oil is even higher at 91 percent. Olive oil is high on the monounsaturated fatty acids list at 77 percent.

Another type of fat that you may have heard about is called trans-fatty acid. This fat doesn't occur naturally. Instead, it is created through hydrogenation, a manufacturing process that changes vegetable oils into semi-solid compounds. The chemical change trans-fatty acid goes through makes it act more like saturated fat in the body, which means it can also raise blood cholesterol. Lard substitutes and tub and stick margarine are two examples of products that contain trans-fatty acids.

Dawn Says

There's been a lot of controversy over trans-fatty acids in recent years. Research has shown that products that contain them can have negative effects on blood cholesterol levels. Some studies also point to higher incidences of breast cancer among women who use these products. When it comes to protecting your heart health, however, fats derived from plants are still a better choice than those that come from animals. If you're going to use them in solid form, be sure to choose those that are labeled as having no trans-fatty acids. Also limit your exposure to trans-fatty acids by avoiding processed baked goods, which usually contain a fair amount of the stuff.

Many people believe that all fat that is ingested is stored as fat in the body, but this isn't true. (If you eat too much fat, however, it is easily converted to stored body fat, so balance is key.) When you eat fat, enzymes in your small intestine rearrange it into new, smaller triglycerides. These smaller particles are then absorbed by your small intestine and combined with small amounts of other substances to form *lipoproteins* called chylomicrons. These circulate in your bloodstream and deliver the triglycerides to your cells, where they can be put to use immediately or stored.

Triglycerides that are stored in the body's fat tissues are calories waiting to be called into action. They also store essential fatty acids, or EFAs, which are essential to some of the body's most basic and important functions, such as growth, reproduction, and skin maintenance, but which it can't make on its own.

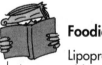

Foodie

Lipoproteins are a combination of fat and protein that transport lipids in the blood.

Common Dietary Sources of Lipids

Food	Percent Fat Saturated	Percent Unsaturated	Percent
Animal Sources			
Beef	16–42	52	48
Butter	81	55	36
Chicken	10–17	30	70

continues

Common Dietary Sources of Lipids (continued)

Food	Percent Fat Saturated	Percent Unsaturated	Percent
Ham, sliced	23	45	55
Lamb	19–29	60	40
Pork	32	45	55
Veal cutlet	10	50	50
Plant Sources			
Carrot	0	0	0
Cashews	48	18	82
Corn oil	100	7	78
Cottonseed oil	100	21.5	71.5
Margarine	81	26	66
Olive oil	100	14	86
Peanut butter	50	25	75
Potato chips	35	25	75
Soybean oil	100	14	71.5

From: McArdle, Katch, and Katch. Sports & Exercise Nutrition.

All About Omegas

In recent years, certain types of fatty acids became dietary darlings after studies showed that they could actually be good for us. For centuries, indigenous people in the Arctic have eaten large amounts of fat harvested from the animals that comprise the majority of their diet—seal, whale, and fish. However, rather than suffering from fat-related health problems, they instead enjoyed extremely good health.

In studies of Greenland Eskimos, researchers found that the fat from these animals contained two types of polyunsaturated fat, and that this fat could protect against heart disease. Several other studies since then have confirmed what the previous researchers had found. In one, heart attacks in men who ate at least 7 ounces of fish a week were reduced 42 percent over men who rarely ate fish. What's more, the study showed that the men benefited from eating fish on a regular basis even if they had other health risks that could affect their hearts. Furthermore, heart attack survivors who were given one gram of fish oil daily for more than three years had lower rates of sudden cardiac death and overall cardiac mortality than those who did not take the supplement.

Known as omega-3s, these fats are found primarily in the oils of cold-water fish, shellfish, and sea mammals.

Dawn Says
Fish oil has proven to be so beneficial to heart health that the American Heart Association now recommends a diet rich in it. The chances of your chowing down on a whale or a seal are probably pretty slim, but you can get health-promoting omega-3s from eating oily, cold-water fish like tuna, herring, sardines, and mackerel on a regular basis—at least once or twice a week. Better yet, and a good option if you're a vegetarian or you simply don't like to eat fish, is taking fish oil supplements daily.

Omega-3s can also be found—in varying quantities—in some nuts and seeds (flaxseed, hemp seed, soybeans, and walnuts) and in the oils derived from them. It's also possible to add omega-3s to your diet by eating dark, leafy vegetables. You can also buy special eggs that have high omega-3 levels, which come from chickens that eat algae along with their chicken feed.

Omega-3 isn't the only omega fat that you need to know about, but it's the most important one, as well as the one that takes a little work when it comes to ensuring that you get enough of it. Omega-6 is another omega fat to keep an eye out for, because it's an important source of linoleic acid, an essential fatty acid that is also vital to good health. However, it's pretty easy to get enough omega-6 since it is contained in many seeds and nuts and a number of vegetable oils, including corn, grapeseed, peanut, soybean, and sunflower. It's also found in the fat of animals—pigs and poultry among them—that are raised on corn.

The Cholesterol Connection

Up to now we've referred to cholesterol in passing a couple of times, so you've probably figured out that there's a connection between it and fat. There definitely is, and we'll get to what that connection is in a moment. First, let's take a closer look at what cholesterol is.

Cholesterol is, simply, a hard, waxy, fatlike substance. It can be found in all parts of the body, including the nervous system, muscles, skin, liver, intestines, and heart. It belongs to a class of molecules called steroids and it exists only in animal tissue. It is a lipid, but it's not the same kind of lipid that we've been discussing, as it differs chemically from triglycerides. Your liver also produces cholesterol and it makes all you'll ever need of the stuff. Even if you never ate any foods that contain cholesterol, you'd still have some in your body.

Like fat, cholesterol gets a bum rap for its well-publicized role in promoting heart disease. And, just like fat, the vital role it plays in the body is also largely overshadowed because of it. Just take a look at all the things that cholesterol does:

- It forms and maintains cell membranes.

- It enables the formation of the sex hormones progesterone, testosterone, estradiol, and cortisol.

- It assists the production of bile salts, which help to digest food.

- It helps form tissues, organs, and body structures during fetal development.

- It assists the synthesis of vitamin D.

Gives you a little more respect for the stuff, doesn't it?

Plant foods contain no cholesterol, but it's found in abundance in animal foods, especially egg yolks, red meat, and organ meats. Shellfish also contains a relatively large amount of cholesterol, as do dairy products such as whole milk, ice cream, butter, and cream cheese.

"Good" vs. "Lousy" Cholesterol

Cholesterol combines with two different types of lipoproteins that transport it in your body. LDL, or low-density lipoprotein, is what we call bad, or "lousy" cholesterol. It consists of 75 percent cholesterol and comprises the majority of the cholesterol circulating in your blood. You want some LDL in your system, as it's necessary for delivering cholesterol to the parts of your body that need it. However, too much LDL causes the cholesterol to build up in the walls of your arteries. Once it's there, it damages the sensitive lining of the arteries, eventually leading to hardening of the arteries.

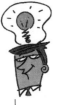

Eat It Up!

LDL lipoprotein is called "low-density" because it has less protein than other lipoproteins.

High-density lipoprotein, which we commonly call "good" cholesterol, contains far more protein than cholesterol and comprises only about 20 to 30 percent of the total cholesterol in your blood. Unlike LDL, HDL has a positive impact on your body because it removes cholesterol from the artery walls and takes it to the liver, where it is incorporated into bile and removed from your body through your intestinal tract.

Now, here's the connection between fat and cholesterol. Saturated fat can raise blood cholesterol levels and clog up arteries even more. When you eat food that is high in animal fat, you're delivering a one-two punch to your circulatory system since they contain both saturated fat and cholesterol.

Cholesterol by the Numbers

The amount of cholesterol in the body is measured through a blood test called a serum lipid profile. The results of that test are represented in several ways:

- Total cholesterol, which, as the term suggests, is a measurement of both types of cholesterol. According to the American Heart Association, for adults, anything less than 200 mg/dL is considered desirable. Levels in the 200 to 239 mg/dL range are considered borderline high risk. Anything over 240 mg/dL is considered high risk.

- HDL cholesterol (the good stuff). In men, the average is 50 to 60 mg/dL; in women, the average range is from 50 to 60 mg/dL. The higher the number, the better. Anything less than 40 mg/dL is considered too low.

- LDL cholesterol (the bad stuff). In adults, this number should be from less than 100 mg/dL to 129 mg/dL, with less than 100 mg/dL being optimal.

- Cholesterol ratio. This is the total cholesterol divided by HDL. It's desirable to keep the ratio below 5:1. The optimum ratio is 3.5:1.

Dawn Says
Even if you're perfectly healthy and show no signs of problems related to high LDL cholesterol, it's a good idea to have a serum lipid profile done every couple of years or so.

Triglycerides are also measured in a serum lipid test. For these, levels less than 150 mg/dL are considered normal, 150–199 mg/dL is borderline high, 200–499 mg/dL is high, and 500 mg/dL or higher is very high.

Checking Cholesterol Content

Dietary fat and cholesterol are listed as two separate categories on food nutrition labels, so it's pretty easy to know how much of each you're eating when you're relying on prepackaged products. But here's where a lot of people go wrong when choosing foods based on cholesterol and fat levels: They think that food with labels that state "no cholesterol" also have no fat. As you can see by the following chart, however, they're dead wrong about that. Mayonnaise doesn't have much cholesterol because it's made from vegetable oil, but it's almost entirely fat.

Cholesterol Content of Some Common Foods

Food	Quantity	Cholesterol, mg
Meat		
Brains, pan fried	3 oz.	1,696
Liver, chicken	3 oz.	537
Caviar	3 oz.	497
Liver, beef, fried	3 oz.	410
Spare ribs, cooked	6 oz.	198
Shrimp, boiled	3 oz.	166
Tuna, light, water-packed	1 can	93
Chicken breast, fried, no skin	3 oz.	91
Halibut, smoked	3 oz.	86
Lambchop, broiled	1	84
Abalone, fried	3 oz.	80
Hamburger patty	3 oz.	75
Corned beef	3 oz.	73
Chicken or turkey, light meat	3 oz.	70
Lobster, cooked	3 oz.	61
Clams	3 oz.	57
Taco, beef	1	57
Swordfish, broiled	3 oz.	50
Bacon strips	3 pieces	36
Hot dog	1	29
Hot dog, beef	1	27
French fries, MacDonald's	regular	13
Dairy		
Egg salad	1 cup	629
Custard, baked	1 cup	213
Egg, yolk	1 large	211
Ice cream, soft-serve, vanilla	1 cup	153
Eggnog	1 cup	149

Food	Quantity	Cholesterol, mg
Ice cream, rich	1 cup	88
Pizza, cheese	1 slice	47
Milk, whole	1 cup	34
Cottage cheese, large curd	1 cup	34
Cheese, cheddar	1 oz.	30
Milk, low-fat, 2%	1 cup	18
Chocolate milkshake	1 cup	13
Butter	1 pat	11
Cottage cheese, low-fat 1%	1 cup	10
Yogurt, low-fat with fruit	1 cup	10
Buttermilk (<1% fat)	1 cup	5
Mayonnaise	1 TB.	5

Source: McArdle

"No cholesterol" also doesn't necessarily mean "low calorie." Sugar is often added to low-fat/low-cholesterol products to make up for the satisfaction factor that these products often lack. Compare a low-fat/low-cholesterol product with its high-fat counterpart (lots of crackers come both ways). You'll probably see more sugar products in the low-fat version.

Keeping Fat and Cholesterol in Check

As previously mentioned, just about everyone can stand to trim some fat from his or her diet. While there is no set standard for optimal fat intake for either the general population or for athletes, most health professionals recommend keeping fat intake at about 30 percent of your total calories, with only 10 percent or less of the fat you eat coming from saturated sources. The American Heart Association recommends eating no more than 300 mg a day of cholesterol. Reducing the amount of food you eat that contains saturated fat is an easy way to keep both fat and cholesterol levels under control.

The Least You Need to Know

♦ Fat is a vital macronutrient and an essential source of energy for athletes.

♦ All types of fat can cause health problems when eaten in excess.

♦ Saturated fat can both increase blood cholesterol and promote heart disease.

♦ Low-fat is a good way to go, but a diet too low in fat can cause vitamin deficiencies and other health problems.

Watering It Down: The Importance of H_2O

In This Chapter

- ◆ Hydration basics
- ◆ How your body uses fluids
- ◆ Recognizing the signs of dehydration
- ◆ Best water alternatives

Of all the nutrients known to humankind, water—one of the most common substances in the world—is the most important. When people don't drink enough water, all sorts of ugly things start to happen. Go without it long enough, and you'll die. Water, in fact, is ranked second only to oxygen as being essential for sustaining life.

There are lots of things you can do from a nutritional point of view to enhance your athletic performance, but staying well hydrated—that is, drinking enough water—will make the greatest impact. So grab a glass of the clear stuff and drink up!

Water, Water, Everywhere

Water is important because it can comprise nearly three quarters of our body mass—between 40 to 70 percent in adults, and even a higher percentage in children. Every tissue and organ in the body depends on water that is inside the cells (*intracellular*) or surrounding the cells (*extracellular*) to function correctly. Water's role in the body includes the following:

◆ Transporting nutrients and oxygen throughout the body

◆ Converting food into energy

◆ Regulating body temperature

◆ Flushing out toxins and body wastes

◆ Moistening the tissues of the eyes, nose, and mouth

◆ Cushioning and lubricating joints and internal organs

◆ Assisting the passage of substances between cells and blood vessels

Foodie

Intracellular refers to water that is found inside the cells in the body. **Extracellular** refers to fluids surrounding the cells.

The majority of the water contained in the body—about 62 percent—is intracellular. The rest is extracellular. Extracellular water is further divided into two categories—intravascular, or the fluid found in the circulatory system (blood plasma), and interstitial, which is found between the cells in the eyes, lymph glands, spinal cord, saliva—basically everywhere there is extracellular water that isn't part of the circulatory system. The fluid you lose when you sweat primarily comes from blood plasma, which accounts for around 20 percent of your extracellular fluid.

Dawn Says

On a normal day, doing regular activities, you lose about 96 ounces of water—about 4 to 8 ounces from the soles of your feet, 16 ounces from perspiration, 48 ounces in your urine, and 16 to 32 ounces from breathing. This means that your body's water supply has to be replenished on a regular basis. And we're not talking about just a couple of ounces of fluid here—the average person has to take in 2½ quarts, or 90 ounces, of water every day to replace what is lost. People who expend more energy than others—for example, athletes—need even more than this.

Research has found that people who are well hydrated simply function more effectively. They also have higher metabolic rates, resist colds and infections more easily, and are less likely to feel tired during the day.

Being adequately hydrated also makes a big difference in whether muscles are being built up or broken down. In other words, it takes water to make muscle. In cells that are well volumized—meaning that they have a healthy amount of water in them—optimal protein synthesis can take place because more nutrients can enter the cells. Dehydration, on the other hand, causes muscle breakdown as it hampers protein synthesis and stimulates muscle-destroying hormones. Seeing bodybuilders walking around with jugs of water makes sense now, doesn't it?

Water also plays a big role in regulating weight. In fact, if you need to lose weight, water is your best friend. Not only does drinking more water help stave off hunger pangs, it also helps you burn fat. As you'll read more about, further on in this chapter, the kidneys filter and remove waste products that are in your body. If you're dehydrated, they have a tough time doing their job effectively, so they ask your liver to help out. One of the liver's functions is to burn fat, which it can't do as well when it's working overtime to assist stressed-out kidneys. So less body fat is metabolized and more is stored, resulting in weight gain or a weight-loss plateau.

How Dry I Am

The opposite of hydration is dehydration, and, unfortunately, it's the latter state that far too many of us walk around in on a regular basis. Not only does time spent indoors in dry, artificially heated or cooled environments rob us of precious moisture, we drink far too many beverages that contain caffeine and alcohol, both proven diuretics that rob the body of water. Combine the two and you have a population that is chronically running low on fluids.

Some of your hydration needs are met by what you eat. Fruits and vegetables, and especially lettuce, cantaloupe, watermelon, celery, cucumbers, and broccoli, contain fair amounts of water—up to 90 percent in some cases. Your body also produces water when it turns food molecules into energy, which provides about 25 percent of the daily water requirement of a sedentary person. The rest of your daily water requirement must be ingested in liquid form. However, most people don't drink nearly enough fluids of any type, and they're far from drinking

Eat It Up!

An estimated 75 percent of Americans are chronically dehydrated.

enough water, which is the best of all of them. When you're low on water, your body will protect essential tissues and organs by taking water from other parts of your system. The result is a laundry list of problems ranging from headaches and fatigue to tissue damage and hypertension.

The FDA Water Chart.

(FDA)

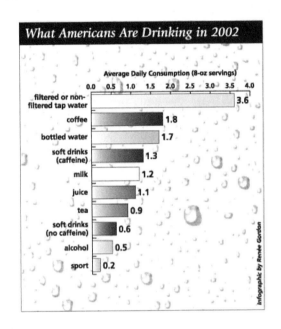

Other problems linked to low water intake include:

♦ Kidney damage. As previously mentioned, wastes such as uric acid, urea, and lactic acid all have to be dissolved in the water in your blood before the kidneys can remove them. When you're dehydrated, your blood plasma level goes down and the kidneys have to work harder, which can result in incomplete removal of wastes—in other words, your blood gets dirty—and kidney damage.

♦ Joint problems. The cartilage at the ends of long bones and between the vertebrae of the spine have a substance called synovial fluid in it, which lubricates the joints when they move. Water is the primary substance that makes up this fluid. The surfaces of the joints can move freely when cartilage is well hydrated. If the cartilage is dehydrated, the joints can't move as smoothly. Over time, this causes joint deteriorization, pain, and loss of mobility.

- Muscle weakness. The cells in your muscles need electrolytes—mineral salts such as calcium, magnesium, sodium, and potassium—to work properly. These substances can't get into the cells without first being dissolved in water. When water levels are low, it's harder for the electrolytes to get in, which makes it more difficult for your muscles to contract. In certain activities, such as sprints and short-distance swimming, one second of difficulty in this arena can mean the difference between first place and tenth place.

- Digestive problems. Digesting solid foods takes a lot of water. If you don't drink enough, the acids and enzymes in your stomach can't do their job as well. In addition, the lack of adequate water in the stomach concentrates those acids and enzymes, causing heartburn and gastritis.

- Impaired brain function. Brain tissue contains the most water of any part of the body at around 85 percent. When fluid levels drop, it simply can't function as well. If you lose as little as 2 percent of your overall body weight through dehydration, your ability to track an object decreases by 20 percent. If you're a tennis or basketball player, this could be lethal to your game. Early symptoms of dehydration include headaches and lethargy. Stay dehydrated long enough, and you run the risk of delirium, seizures, and brain damage.

Many people mistake the physical symptoms of dehydration, such as headaches and fatigue, as hunger pangs. Because all food contains a certain amount of liquid, eating will slake these feelings to some extent, but it really doesn't solve the underlying problem. Substituting food for water when dehydrated also adds calories to the diet that are often not needed, no matter how healthy the source. Take in too little water and your body will also start retaining the water it does have to compensate for the shortage.

Eat It Up!

Back pain is another indication that you're not getting enough water. Almost three quarters of the weight in the upper body is supported by water contained in the spine. And, the spine relies on water stored in the discs between its joints to function properly. When water levels are low, the discs lose their ability to absorb shocks to the spine, resulting in pain.

Taking the Heat

Dehydration also contributes to heat-related illnesses, which are a particular concern for athletes. As mentioned earlier in this chapter, water plays an important role in the body's thermoregulatory system, which, as the name implies, is what allows the body to heat and cool itself as necessary.

The part of the brain called the hypothalamus is what controls body temperature. In effect, it works like an automatic thermostat. It's set to a certain temperature— 98.6 degrees, more or less. When it senses heat gain or loss either from temperature changes in the blood or from heat sensors in the skin, it tells the body how to respond so it can maintain its preset temperature. Unlike a thermostat, however, the hypothalamus only governs the body's physical reaction to being too hot or too cold. It can't turn off the body's internal combustion engine.

The body's thermoregulation system primarily protects against overheating as it's more of a problem than being too cold is. No matter where we are or what our activity level is, we're always generating energy. If that energy was allowed to build up in the body, our core temperatures would go up too high and we could die.

Evaporation is the body's main defense against overheating. When the body starts to heat up, the sweat glands secrete large quantities of hypotonic saline solution—what we call sweat, which is mostly water. When sweat reaches the skin, it evaporates and brings the skin's temperature down. As the skin cools, blood temperature goes down with it.

Eat It Up! _____

The body loses heat through other mechanisms as well, including radiation, conduction, and convection. But evaporation through the skin and respiratory passages is the body's main physiological response to overheating.

Most of the time conditions are such that thermoregulation can take place as it's supposed to. However, your thermoregulation system can quickly become overloaded when you're working out or training, especially when it's done at high levels of intensity. As the body's core temperature rises, perspiration increases as well. If the fluids lost through sweat aren't replenished on a regular basis, the body becomes dehydrated and can't produce enough sweat to cool itself off.

When this happens, heat-related problems can surface extremely quickly. Cramps and dizziness are the problems that erupt first. While of concern in and of themselves, they often are indications that more serious problems, including heat exhaustion and heatstroke, are just around the corner.

Working out in hot and humid conditions, as many athletes do, causes even more problems. As humidity rises, sweat can't evaporate as efficiently. When the weather is hot, the body can heat up even higher as it also absorbs heat from the sun and from hard surfaces such as concrete and asphalt. Since 1995, at least 20 high school, college, and professional football players have died from hyperthermia, or high body heat, when they overheated during practice or competition. Korey Stringer, the

Minnesota Vikings offensive tackle who died in 2001 after he collapsed following a practice session in the brutal heat and humidity of a Minnesota summer, had an internal temperature of 108.8—10 degrees higher than normal and a level that's fatal in 80 percent of heat-related cases. High body heat and dehydration were also linked to the deaths of three college-level wrestlers during 1997.

Eat It Up! _____

Heatstroke is ranked third behind head and neck trauma and cardiac disorders as a cause of death among high school athletes in the United States.

Sweating the Cold

Athletes who compete in the water and the cold also aren't off the hook when it comes to heat-related illnesses. They can happen in more moderate conditions as well, which is why it's important to stay on top of water intake no matter where you are. Swimmers may not feel like they're sweating when they're in the water, but they actually lose fluid at about the same rate as runners do. In fact, being in the water stimulates body water loss through increased urine production. It may seem strange to have to gulp down water when you're surrounded by it, but that's exactly what you have to do if you participate in water sports.

It's important to remember that you're always losing water—even when it's cold out and the sun isn't shining—which means that you have to be vigilant about replacing it. You may be more aware of the physical cues of dehydration when it's warm out, but you need just as many fluids when the weather is cold. When temperatures drop, your body also has to expend more energy just to stay warm. This means you'll lose fluids even more rapidly, and because it's cold, you won't be as aware of the fact that you're sweating.

Diving In

We've been preaching the water gospel pretty heavily up to now and for good reason. Unless you're one of those rare birds who really focus on keeping your hydration levels in balance, chances are very good that you're dehydrated to some degree. If you're not sure that you fall into this category, there's a very simple way to test yourself. All you have to do is check the color of your urine. Yes, it's a little ooky, but it's one of the best ways to tell if you're getting enough water. If it's light in color and odor, you're in the clear. Dark, strong-smelling urine is a sure sign of dehydration. Other signs that you should be drinking more water include:

◆ A sore throat, dry cough, or hoarseness

◆ Burning in your stomach

◆ Muscle cramps

◆ Headaches

Staying well hydrated means drinking lots of water and drinking it often, whether you're thirsty or not. In fact, it's important to drink before you feel thirsty because a substantial amount of dehydration can occur before the sensation of thirst arises.

How much do you need to drink? The general rule of thumb is 64 ounces of water a day, which equates to eight eight-ounce glasses (two quarts), plus additional water for workouts. How much extra depends on a variety of factors, including what you eat (diets that are heavy on protein require more water to remove wastes), how strenuously you're exercising, the conditions in which you're working out, and other factors. You'll find more information on how to determine how much more water you should drink, and when you should drink it, in Chapter 3.

Working It In

If you're not used to quaffing much water, the thought of gulping down two quarts of water a day can be daunting. However, it really isn't all that much. If you drink an eight-ounce glass of water with each main meal, you're already at 24 ounces, almost half of your minimum requirement. Here are some other ways to up your water intake:

◆ Begin and end the day with water. Your body loses water when you're asleep, so be sure to drink a glass of water before bedtime and when you wake up.

◆ Bring a supply of bottled water with you when shopping, traveling, or exercising— winter or summer.

◆ If you drink a lot of fruit juice, try cutting your juice with water to a 50/50 concentration.

◆ Substitute herbal tea for caffeinated drinks. Since it's not caffeinated, it counts toward your daily water requirement. Make sure, however, that you choose teas that contain no caffeine. Some herbal teas do, so read labels carefully.

Until your body adjusts to its increased fluid levels, you may need to visit the bathroom more often. If you spread out your water intake over the course of your waking hours, however, you shouldn't be too uncomfortable. The human body can only absorb about a quart of water per hour, and it does a better job of absorbing it if you drink it in small amounts instead of thirst-quenching gulps, so you'll actually stay better hydrated if you pace yourself. If you're worried about a full bladder waking you up from a sound sleep, get the majority of your water in before 7 P.M.

Food Foul-Ups

The day before an important race or event is not the time to start a rehydration program. Starting well before them will give your body time to adjust to increased fluid levels and minimize your need for rest breaks.

Best Water Choices

Water is water is water, right? Wrong! Depending on where you live, the water that comes out of your tap may or may not be the best choice for drinking. Now, before we go much further, be assured that the water in most communities is perfectly safe to drink. If you live in an area where your water is municipally supplied, check with your local water board to see what's actually in the stuff you're drinking. If your water comes from other sources, such as from a private well, you can have it analyzed if you're at all concerned about it.

> **Dawn Says**
>
> Water can get contaminated in a variety of ways, ranging from fertilizer runoff to lead leaching from old pipes. When it comes to such a vital nutrient, it's better to be safe than sorry. If you're concerned at all about the water where you live, get it tested.

From the Bottle

Bottled water is today a hugely popular alternative to tap water. However, beyond its taste and color, most of it isn't much different than the stuff that comes out of your tap at home. In fact, many bottled waters are exactly that—tap water that's been filtered.

Bottled water is regulated by the U.S. Food and Drug Administration, which sets specific regulations to ensure that the bottled water we buy is safe. However, because the FDA uses the Environmental Protection Agency's standards regarding contaminants, contaminant levels in bottled and tap water are similar. What bottled water generally contains less of is lead. On the other hand tap water that is municipally supplied usually contains fluoride, which is added to promote strong teeth and prevent tooth decay.

Bottled water, especially if it's distilled or purified through reverse osmosis, generally doesn't contain fluoride, although some brands do add it. Small children who drink bottled water that doesn't have fluoride added to it may need supplemental fluoride to make sure their teeth stay healthy.

Filtering It

Putting a water filter on your main tap or buying a container filtration system are other alternatives to drinking your tap water straight. Both methods remove the majority of impurities and contaminants that tap water can contain. They also remove most of the objectionable smells, color, and tastes often present in municipal water. Filtering your own water is usually cheaper than buying bottled water as well.

Variations on the Water Theme

As this chapter stresses, water is the single best choice for keeping your body hydrated. It's widely available, cheap, and calorie-free—all factors that put it at the top of the hydration list. When you're exercising, however, it's not the only choice. Sports drinks with a 5 to 8 percent carbohydrate solution are another option, albeit a much more expensive one. Studies show that water is the best choice for rehydration for activities lasting less than an hour. After this, sports drinks help replenish fluid, electrolytes, and a small amount of needed energy. Beyond this, sports drinks simply taste better to some, so people are apt to drink more of them than they are of water.

Designer waters are the newest fad in the hydration arena. There are a variety of specialty waters now available, with more of them hitting the market all the time. Like sports drinks, some contain electrolytes that can help speed hydration. Others contain added vitamins, minerals, and even herbs or caffeine. Still others are engineered in various ways that are thought to enhance their qualities and benefits, and, in turn, enhance your performance. All are expensive options compared to plain water.

Is designer water worth the price? Probably not, but if you believe that it will make you run faster or jump higher, it might. You're better off saving your money and spending it on healthy food … and maybe a new water bottle so you can take some of the wet stuff with you wherever you go.

The Least You Need to Know

◆ Maintaining adequate hydration levels means drinking lots of water and drinking it often, whether you're thirsty or not.

◆ You're always losing water, which means that you have to be vigilant about replacing it.

◆ Plain old water from the tap is usually safe, although it might smell or taste funny.

◆ Designer water might deliver some nutritional benefit above and beyond that of plain water, but it's not worth the added expense.

Chapter 11

Vital Vitamins and Mighty Minerals

In This Chapter

- Understanding vitamins and minerals
- RDAs vs. DRIs
- Best vitamin and mineral sources
- All about antioxidants

Walk into just about any grocery store, drug store, or mass-market retailer, and you'll see them: row upon row of bottles containing vitamins and minerals in all shapes, sizes, dosages, and formulations. Multivitamins, B-complex vitamins, chelated minerals, stress-relief formula, men's formula, women's formula, antioxidants—it's enough to boggle your mind!

The role that these nutrients play in good health has been known for some time now, but only in the last 20 years or so has vitamin and mineral supplementation really taken off. If you're wondering what all the hoopla is about, stay tuned. We'll give you the lowdown on what you need to know about the vitamin and mineral scene.

Small but Mighty

Vitamins and minerals—called micronutrients in nutritional lingo—are the substances your body needs to put the macronutrients you eat to work. They don't contain energy of their own, but they are essential for releasing energy from your food. They also play a key role in tissue growth, healing, and repair.

> ## Eat It Up!
>
> In 1911, Casimir Funk, a Polish scientist, combined the Latin word *vita*, meaning "life," and *amine*, an organic compound derived from ammonia, to create a new word that described the substances in food that could prevent such diseases as beri-beri, scurvy, and pellagra. The term "vitamine" was later shortened to vitamin when research showed that not all vitamins were amines. Vitamins and minerals are called micronutrients because you need much less of them than the macronutrients—protein, carbohydrates, and fat.

Vitamins and minerals are big news today for several reasons. First, we know a great deal more about how they work and their importance in maintaining good health. Second, there is a greater need for taking supplemental vitamins and minerals than ever before. Experts used to believe that we could get all the vitamins and minerals we needed if we just followed a balanced diet and ate the right amount of food. The problem is, most people don't do either of these things.

Research has shown that many of the foods we eat don't contain the same levels of vitamins and minerals that they once did. It is difficult, if not impossible, to eat enough of some of these foods to meet the recommended daily requirements for certain vitamins, not to mention the higher levels needed of some micronutrients for protection against chronic and degenerative illnesses.

Even doctors and other health experts who were once staunchly against vitamin and mineral supplementation are now strongly in favor of it. Taking your vitamins (and minerals) is now seen as an essential component of a nutritionally sound diet.

There are 13 vitamins and about 22 minerals that you need to keep your body operating the way it should. A reference system called the Dietary Reference Intakes, or DRI, determines how much of these substances we need for basic good health.

All About Daily Values

The first set of recommendations for vitamin and mineral consumption was published more than 60 years ago by the Food and Nutrition Board of the National Academy of Sciences. Called the Recommended Dietary Allowances (RDAs), these guidelines made recommendations for nutrient intake levels that experts believed would meet the nutritional needs for most healthy people and were based on research that was available at the time.

The primary goal of the RDA guidelines was to prevent diseases like beriberi, rickets, scurvy, and pellagra that are caused by vitamin deficiencies. While the guidelines were useful, they were designed to meet the needs of large groups of people rather than individuals. Statistics showed that getting the recommended levels of RDAs would keep the majority of people healthy. However, no one knew if the RDAs would meet the nutritional needs of specific individuals.

In the years that followed, considerably more research took place on vitamins and minerals. Much more was now known about the roles they played in promoting good health, and what happened when people didn't get enough of them (or got too much of them). As a result of this data, the FNB redefined nutrient requirements and developed specific recommendations for both groups and individuals.

The Dietary Reference Intakes (DRIs) are similar to the older RDAs, but they do a better job of taking into account the different nutritional needs of various populations. As such, they provide several values for each nutrient instead of just one. The new values are also based more on the philosophy of preventing chronic diseases instead of preventing nutritional deficiencies.

The DRI system is multilevel, meaning that it offers guidelines for both recommended and maximum intake amounts. It uses the following reference values:

Eat It Up!

The new DRI system is a joint effort being undertaken by the National Academy of Sciences in the United States and Health Canada, the Canadian equivalent of the NAS. The system will eventually replace both the RDA system in the United States and Canada's Recommended Nutrient Intake (RNI) system.

◆ Recommended Dietary Allowance (RDA). This is the intake level that meets the nutrient needs of almost all healthy individuals in specific age and gender groups. This is the basic reference value to use when determining the levels of various nutrients you need in your diet.

- Estimated Average Requirement (EAR). This is the nutrient level determined to meet the needs of 50 percent of individuals in a specific group. It is based on strong research evidence and is used to determine a nutrient's RDA.

- Adequate Intake (AI). Adequate intake is set when there isn't enough data to establish an RDA. These figures are less precise than RDAs, but will still meet or exceed the nutrient needs for almost all healthy people.

- Tolerable Upper limit (UL). This is the highest vitamin or mineral level that can be safely taken without risking adverse health effects. It can't be set for all nutrients due to the lack of scientific information for some of them.

These terms can be a bit confusing. However, the important ones to know about are RDA and AI, which together form the basis for basic good health. These days, you'll see the abbreviation DV, for Daily Value, used in place of RDA on many nutritional labels.

The charts here show the current RDA (also called RDI for Reference Daily Intake, or DRV for Daily Reference Value, or just DV for Daily Value) for adults, along with the highest DRI and the upper limit for each nutrient.

Vitamin Intake Levels for Adults

Vitamin	Current RDI	New DRI	UL
A	5000 IU	900 mcg (3000 IU)	3000 mcg (10,000 IU)
C	60 mg	90 mg	2000 mg
D	400 IU (10 mcg)	15 mcg (600 IU)	50 mcg (2000 IU)
E	30 IU (20 mg)	15 mg	1000 mg
K	80 mcg	120 mcg	ND (not determined)
Thiamin	1.5 mg	1.2 mg	ND
Riboflavin	1.7 mg	1.3 mg	ND
Niacin	20 mg	16 mg	35 mg
Vitamin B-6	2 mg	1.7 mg	100 mg
Folate	400 mcg	400 mcg from food, 200 mcg synthetic	1000 mcg synthetic
Vitamin B-12	6 mcg	2.4 mcg	ND
Biotin	300 mcg	30 mcg	ND

Vitamin	Current RDI	New DRI	UL
Pantothenic acid	10 mg	5 mg	ND
Choline	Not establ.	550 mg	3500 mg

Source: Council for Responsible Nutrition

The FNB also set new guidelines for mineral consumption. They are as follows:

Mineral Intake Levels for Adults

Mineral	Current RDI	New DRI	UL
Calcium	1000 mg	1300 mg	2500 mg
Iron	18 mg	18 mg	45 mg
Phosphorus	1000 mg	1250 mg	4000 mg
Iodine	150 mcg	150 mcg	1100 mcg
Magnesium	400 mg	420 mg	350 mg
Zinc	15 mg	11 mg	40 mg
Selenium	70 mcg	55 mcg	400 mcg
Copper	2 mg	0.9 mg	10 mg
Manganese	2 mg	2.3 mg	11 mg
Chromium	120 mcg	35 mcg	ND
Molybdenum	75 mcg	45 mcg	2000 mcg

Source: Council for Responsible Nutrition

Keep in mind that these figures represent only the nutrient levels that have been established to meet basic health needs. Current research has shown that taking in higher levels of certain vitamins and minerals is necessary to prevent many chronic and degenerative diseases. We'll get into more detail about why this is so later in this chapter.

Now that you know a little more about which vitamins and minerals constitute a healthy diet, and how much you should be getting of them on a daily basis, let's take a closer look at what these substances actually do.

Food Foul-Ups

Many people believe in the "more is better" approach when taking vitamin and mineral supplements. However, consuming high levels of some nutrients can actually damage your health and lead to lifelong health problems.

Vital Vitamins

Vitamins are organic substances that play three significant roles in the body: They help it grow, they protect it, and they help regulate its energy. We need 13 vitamins to stay healthy. The human body either can't make these vitamins, or it can't make enough of them. Because of this, we have to get our vitamins from outside sources—the food we eat or the supplements we take.

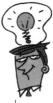

Eat It Up!

The human body can make vitamin D, which is manufactured in the skin when it is exposed to sunlight.

Eat It Up!

Vitamins are a twentieth-century discovery. The first vitamin to be isolated was vitamin A in 1913. Vitamin B12, the most recent vitamin to be discovered, was found in 1948.

Vitamins come in two forms:

- Fat-soluble (A, E, D, K). These vitamins do not dissolve in water and are stored in the body's fat and liver, where they stay until they're needed. Because the body stores these vitamins, taking too much of them can be dangerous.

- Water-soluble (B1, B2, B6, B12, niacin, pantothenic acid, folic acid, biotin, and vitamin C). There is no danger of overloading on these vitamins, as they are excreted in the urine if you take too much of them.

We get the majority of the vitamins we need from the food we eat. However, all food is not created equal when it comes to vitamin content. Vitamin levels can differ significantly depending on how the food is grown and where it is grown. How food is shipped, stored, bought, and cooked can also affect nutrient levels.

Vitamin	Functions	Dietary Sources
Fat-Soluble		
A	Vision, mucous membrane formation, bone and tooth growth, growth and repair of body structure, healthy skin, immune function	Dark green and deep orange vegetables, beef liver, fortified milk, cheese, egg yolks
D (calciferol)	Promotes bone growth and health. Increases calcium and phosphorus absorption	Cod liver oil, eggs, dairy products, fortified milk, and margarine
E (tocopherol)	Antioxidant, prevents cell damage, anticcoagulant	Seeds, nuts, green leafy vegetables, margarines, shortenings, wheat germ

Vitamin	Functions	Dietary Sources
K (phylloquinone)	Blood clotting, involved in glycogen formation	Liver, green leafy vegetables, small amounts in cereals, fruit, meats, milk, yogurt
Water-Soluble		
B1 (thiamine)	Energy metabolism, nervous system function, muscle tone, heart function	Pork, organ meats, whole grains, nuts, legumes, milk, fruits, vegetables, dried yeast
B2 (riboflavin)	Metabolism of carbohydrates, protein, and fat; maintenance of eye tissue, cellular respiration	In many foods, including meats, eggs, milk products, whole-grain and enriched cereal products, wheat germ, green leafy vegetables
B3 (niacin)	Metabolism of carbohydrates, protein, and fat; skin, nervous system and digestive tract health; formation of red blood cells	Milk, eggs, meat, poultry, legumes, peanuts, fish, mushrooms, greens, dried yeast, liver
B6 (pyridoxine)	Protein, carbohydrate, and fatty acid metabolism, red blood cell production, nervous system function, healthy skin	Meats, fish, poultry, vegetables, whole grains, cereals, seeds, dried yeast, organ meats, liver, peanuts, walnuts, dried beans, avocados
Pantothenic acid	Supports adrenal glands, important for healthy skin and nerves, helps metabolize carbohydrates and fats into energy, necessary for making fatty acids, cholesterol, and steroids	Widely available in meat, fish, poultry, milk products, legumes, whole grains; also liver, yeast
Folate (folic acid, folacin)	DNA and RNA synthesis, regulation of growth, breakdown of proteins, maturation of red blood cells, protection against neurological defects in newborns	Legumes, green vegetables, whole-wheat products, meats, eggs, milk product, liver, dried yeast, wheat germ, sweet potatoes
B12 (cobalamin)	Cell synthesis, nerve function, metabolism of carbohydrates, proteins, and fat, formation of red blood cells	Muscle meats, fish, eggs, dairy products

continues

(continued)

Vitamin	Functions	Dietary Sources
Biotin	Fatty acid and carbohydrate metabolism	Legumes, vegetables, meats, liver, egg yolk, nuts, cauliflower, yeast
Vitamin C	Collagen formation, amino acid metabolism, enhanced iron absorption; antioxidant, bone and connective tissue growth, wound repair	Citrus fruits, tomatoes, green peppers, salad greens, potatoes, cabbage, broccoli

To preserve the highest vitamin levels in the foods you eat, follow these guidelines:

1. Avoid wilted or precut items.

2. Avoid soaking vegetables and fruits.

3. Keep peels on when cooking or storing.

4. Prepare vegetables by steaming whenever you can.

5. Cook vegetables quickly at high temperatures.

6. Cook vegetables al dente.

7. Avoid overcooking by making sure that water is at the appropriate temperature before you add food to it.

Danger! Overdose!

As previously mentioned, taking in too much of the fat-soluble vitamins can cause more problems than they solve. While overdosing doesn't happen all that often, it's a good idea to know the symptoms in case you should accidentally ingest more of the following vitamins than you should.

Vitamin	Overdose Level	Symptoms
A	100,000 units/day	Irritability, fatigue, insomnia, bone and joint pain, abnormal bone growth, hair loss, itchy skin, anorexia, decreased blood-clotting time; in children: malaise and fatigue, abnormal growth, pain and tenderness in the long bones, headaches and irritability, flaking of the skin and mucous membranes

Vitamin	Overdose Level	Symptoms
E	Not established (probably high)	Increase in vitamin K requirement
D	4000–10,000 IU/day	Anorexia, nausea, diarrhea, muscular weakness, joint pains, calcification of soft tissues, reabsorption of bone; in children: weakness, lethargy, anorexia, constipation
K	Not established	Gastrointestinal illness, impaired absorption

Boosting Your Energy with the B's

B vitamins are an important part of the Krebs cycle, which is the part of the metabolic process that generates a lot of energy. For this reason, it would seem that taking large doses of this vitamin group would make you feel less fatigued. However, unless you drink too much alcohol on a regular basis, eat a restricted-calorie diet, or eat very high levels of processed, high-fat, high-sugar foods, research suggests that you can meet the minimum requirements for all the B vitamins by eating whole grains, lean meats, lentils, green leafy vegetables, fruits, and milk—in other words, a balanced diet.

Mighty Minerals

Minerals—the inorganic elements that are found in water, topsoil, and beneath the earth's surface—are also essential for good health. Your body requires at least 40 different mineral substances in varying amounts. The key players are the *macrominerals*— seven important substances that your body needs in amounts ranging from a fraction of a gram to several grams.

You need smaller amounts of the second group of minerals, which are called trace minerals or *microminerals*. With these minerals, nutrient levels are measured in milligrams (millionths of a gram) and micrograms (thousandths of a gram). There is even a third classification of minerals known as *microtrace*, ultratrace, or rare earth minerals, which are measured in parts per million (ppm).

 Foodie

Macrominerals are the seven minerals that the body needs large amounts of. Microminerals and microtrace minerals are needed in smaller amounts.

Minerals often play second fiddle to vitamins when micronutrients are discussed, but they really shouldn't. They are just as important as vitamins, and in some respects, even more so. Minerals are what enable vitamins to do their work in the body. Without vitamins, the body can still use minerals. Without minerals, vitamins can do nothing.

Mineral	Function	Dietary Sources
Major		
Calcium	Bone and tooth formation, blood clotting, nerve transmission, smooth muscle contraction	Milk, cheese, dark green vegetables, dried legumes
Chlorine	Important component of extracellular fluids, electrolyte balance	Is part of salt-containing food (see sodium); some vegetables and fruits
Magnesium	Activates enzymes involved in protein synthesis, aids muscle relaxation, helps metabolize carbohydrates and proteins, bone and tooth formation, regulates body temperature	Legumes, nuts, artichokes, avocados, corn, halibut, mackerel, peas, tofu, cocoa, leafy green vegetables, whole-grain cereals and breads, soybeans
Phosphorus	Bone and tooth formation, essential for energy production.	Milk, cheese, yogurt, meat, poultry, grains, fish, legumes, nuts acid-base balance
Potassium	Fluid balance, nerve transmission, carbohydrate metabolism, protein synthesis	Leafy vegetables, cantaloupe, lima beans, potatoes, bananas, milk, meats, coffee, tea, prunes, raisins
Sodium	Acid-base balance, body water balance, nerve function	Common salt, beef, pork, sardines, green olives, sauerkraut, cheese
Sulfur	Acid-base balance, liver function, appears to stabilize protein molecules in the body, especially in the hair, nails, and skin	Present in thiamine, insulin, methionine (essential amino acid) and cysteine (nonessential amino acid); also food preservatives
Minor		
Arsenic	No clear biological function in humans; animal studies indicates a requirement	Dairy products, meat, poultry, fish, grains, cereal

Mineral	Function	Dietary Sources
Boron	Brain function, bone growth, repair, and maintenance	Fruit-based beverages and products, potatoes, legumes, milk, avocado, peanut butter, peanuts
Chromium	Essential for normal sugar and fat metabolism, maintaining normal blood glucose levels	Legumes, cereals, organ meats
Copper	Manufacturing red blood cells, nerves, and collagen; aids iron absorption and transport	Meats, drinking water, nuts, shellfish, organ meats, grains, legumes, dark leafy vegetables
Fluoride	May be important in maintaining bone structure	Drinking water, tea, coffee, seafood
Iodine	Formation of thyroid hormones that regulate metabolism	Seafood, dairy products, vegetables, iodized salt, some drinking water
Iron	Transporting oxygen in bloodstream, immune function, preventing anemia	Eggs, lean meats, legumes, whole grains, green leafy vegetables, soybean flour, prune juice, chicken, tuna
Manganese	Important for skin, bones, menstrual cycle maintenance, and for cholesterol and fatty acids metabolism	Peanuts, pecans, oatmeal, pineapple, juice, some cereals, dried fruits, tea
Molybdenum	Cofactor of several enzymes involved in protein and iron metabolism	Legumes, grain products, cereals, leafy vegetables, nuts
Nickel	No clear biological function established in humans; may support iron absorption or metabolism	Beans, peas, nuts, oatmeal, chocolate
Selenium	Works with vitamin E to protect cells from free radicals	Seafood, meats, milk, eggs, grains
Silicon	No clear biological function in humans identified; thought to play a role in bone function; hair, skin, and fingernail growth	Whole grains, beets, bell peppers, beans, peas

continues

(continued)

Mineral	Function	Dietary Sources
Tin	No biological function in humans identified	Canned foods
Vanadium	Necessary for normal iodine metabolism, thyroid function; no biological function in humans identified	Parsley, black pepper, dill, mushrooms, and shellfish
Zinc	Detoxification of alcohol, boosts immune system, helps maintain healthy skin cells, assists protein digestion, DNA and RNA synthesis, normal insulin activity, wound healing	Shellfish, legumes, organ meat, poultry, pork, seeds, meat, wild rice, wheat germ, yogurt, cashews

Unlike vitamins, minerals can't be destroyed by food handling, processing, cooking, or storage. In fact, you can add iron to your food by cooking in cast-iron skillets, which leach iron into food.

More About Calcium

All minerals are important for your good health, but calcium deserves some special attention. As the most abundant mineral in the body, it combines with phosphorus to build bones and teeth. The calcium in our blood enables our muscles to contract so that we can move and lift weights. It also aids in blood clotting, transmitting nerve impulses, and moving fluids in and out of cells.

Food Foul-Ups

Don't go by blood calcium levels to measure your bone density. If your blood is short on calcium, your body will pull calcium from your bones. For this reason, high levels of blood calcium don't necessarily mean that you have adequate calcium in your bones.

We need calcium throughout our lives to keep our bones strong. However, most adults don't get nearly enough of this important mineral on a daily basis. Part of the problem is that we don't eat enough foods that are high in calcium. However, there are a number of factors that can keep our bodies from absorbing the calcium we do eat, including the following:

- Eating too much protein

- Repetitive alcohol use

- High-fiber foods

- Oxalic acids (contained in some foods)

- Large doses of zinc
- Caffeine
- Aluminum hydroxide (found in some antacids)
- Cigarette smoking
- Nonweight-bearing exercise

Vitamin D increases calcium absorption, which is why milk is fortified with this vitamin. The protein in the milk also stirs up the acid in the stomach and creates a higher amount of calcium absorption.

Eating three to four servings of dairy a day will go a long way toward ensuring adequate calcium levels. So will staying away from alcohol, caffeine, and cigarettes. It's also a good idea to keep an eye on your protein intake and other foods that can interfere with calcium absorption.

If you don't like dairy products, dark green leafy vegetables also contain calcium, but you have to eat a lot of these foods to get enough calcium to meet your daily requirement. Calcium supplementation is often necessary, especially for women, to meet the minimum RDA for this important micronutrient.

More About Iron

Iron is another mineral of special concern to athletes. Iron's main function is to transport oxygen; when iron levels are low there is less oxygen available to the muscles and tissues, and they can't function at normal levels. Strength training, which breaks down muscle tissue and requires a lot of blood-building materials for recovery, can exacerbate iron deficiency. So can aerobic exercise, as the pounding that often accompanies it can break down blood cells, making it difficult to recover from repetitive workouts without eating high-quality proteins.

Athletes who don't eat meat, or who don't eat it very often, run the risk of not having enough iron in their blood. Certain individuals are also at a higher risk of iron deficiency than others. They include these groups:

- Children
- Women who bleed heavily while menstruating
- Pregnant women

Many different animal and plant foods contain iron. However, *heme* iron, which is found in animal protein, is the form that your body prefers, as it can absorb it better. It doesn't do as well with *nonheme* iron, which is found in vegetables, beans, seeds, nuts, and dried fruits (as well as in fortified breads and cereals). You'll have to eat more of these foods to get the same amount of iron provided by animal protein. Or since heme iron increases the amount of nonheme iron absorbed from plant sources, you could eat a little protein along with your plant foods.

All About Antioxidants

Antioxidants are the big news these days. This special group of vitamins and vitamin-like nutrients work to protect the body from harmful molecules called free radicals that impair the human body and cause it to age. Free radicals are caused, interestingly enough, by the oxygen that we use to make energy.

Research has shown that oxygen is both our best friend and our worst enemy. We couldn't live without it, of course, but it can also damage the body from within. Here's how: Our bodies use oxygen to make energy. The byproducts left over from this process—called free radicals—differ from other atoms in the body in that they either are short an electron or have one too many. They're unbalanced, and they will do anything to steal an electron from another atom to balance themselves. When searching for that extra electron, they damage whatever is around them, including the following:

- Cell walls
- Membranes
- Vessels
- The DNA of the cell
- Proteins and fats

Because free radicals are a byproduct of the body's energy-burning process, they are always present in the body. Antioxidants work to keep them in check. However, these little buggers can even duplicate and make more free radicals, thanks to a phenomenon known as oxidative stress, which develops when the free radicals in the body outnumber antioxidants. What's worse, there are numerous other factors outside of the body than can also accelerate free radical growth, including these:

- Pollutants in the water, food, and air

- Ultraviolet rays from the sun

- High stress levels

- Too little or too much exercise

- Poor dietary habits

You read this right. Too much exercise can be just as damaging to your body as too little exercise when it comes to how free radicals affect your system.

What can we do to protect ourselves from free radical damage? We can eat a healthy diet, exercise moderately, and take antioxidants, which stop free radicals in their tracks by providing the electrons they're seeking.

For optimal cell nutrition, it is important to take higher doses of vitamins with antioxidant properties than of the other micronutrients. Doing so will give your body the best defense against degenerative diseases.

There are many different kinds of free radicals, which means that no single antioxidant will wipe them all out. For this reason, it's a good idea to take a variety of antioxidants or a supplement that contains a variety of them. We'll talk about this in more detail in Chapter 14.

 Eat It Up!

Free radicals have also been shown to be a key contributor to many disorders that were once thought to be simply a part of the aging process, such as cancer, rheumatoid arthritis, Alzheimer's disease, heart attacks, and strokes.

To Supplement or Not to Supplement?

There's really no great substitute for the nutrition you get from eating a well-balanced diet. But, for a variety of reasons, very few people achieve optimal micronutrient levels through what they eat. A two-year study of Americans' eating habits conducted by the U.S. Department of Agriculture found that more than 80 percent of women and more than 70 percent of men consumed less than two thirds of the RDA for one or more micronutrients. Fewer than half the participants met the RDAs for vitamins A, B6, and E, or for calcium, magnesium, and zinc.

If you are one of the few who eat perfectly, you might not need a supplement. But there are many factors beyond your control that can decrease the vitamin and mineral levels in your food and increase your need for them. So why take the chance? When it comes to ensuring your good health, the money you spend on a good multivitamin and mineral supplement is well worth it.

Dawn Says
I believe that everyone should take a multivitamin, even children, starting at age 13 months. With our environment as it is today, coupled with poor nutrition and exercise habits, it's almost impossible to get the amount of vitamins and minerals necessary to both fuel cells with optimal nutrition and protect them from damage. It would take some *15,000 calories a day* of the best foods you could possibly eat to do both.

For more on how you can select the best supplements, and on how to read supplement labels, turn to Chapter 14.

The Least You Need to Know

- The human body needs 13 vitamins and about 22 minerals to operate the way it should.

- You can determine your basic vitamin and mineral needs by knowing what the RDA is of each.

- Eating well might provide adequate vitamin and mineral levels. You can ensure that you get enough of them by taking a good multivitamin and mineral supplement.

- Antioxidants—a special group of vitamins and vitaminlike substances—can help prevent degenerative diseases and slow down aging by minimizing the negative affect of free radicals on the body.

Part 3

Hitting the Food Trail

Eating right doesn't just happen. It takes a certain amount of forethought and a good amount of planning ahead to put the right food in your pantry, on your table, and inside of you!

In this part, you'll find handy and practical advice on how to stay on the eating healthy trail both at home and away. You'll learn how to stock your shelves with healthy food choices and how to avoid falling into the traps that can lure you away from your quest for healthy food when you're in the supermarket. You'll also get the inside scoop on what convenience carbohydrates can do for you, along with information on buying vitamins and supplements, on eating on the go, and on eating for optimal performance both before and after your workout, practice, competition, or game.

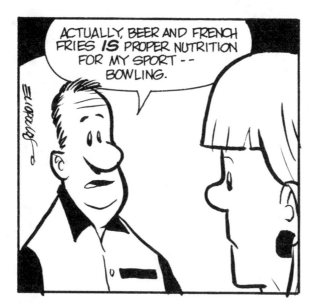

Stocking the Shelves

In This Chapter

◆ Planning your attack

◆ What every kitchen needs

◆ Understanding grocery store layouts

◆ Money-saving tips

By now you've probably realized that healthy eating requires some discipline. It also calls for a certain amount of planning ahead. How many times have you walked into your kitchen in search of a healthy snack, only to come away empty-handed because you couldn't find any?

Want to know a secret? The best way to keep healthy eating on the right track is by having nutritious food on hand at all times. If your refrigerator and pantry are full of healthy choices, you're going to be far less motivated to go out in search of junk food when you're hungry.

When life is busy, meal planning and grocery shopping might seem like more effort than they're worth. However, they're two of the best habits you can get into when it comes to eating for optimum performance. If the mere mention of the word "plan" makes your toes curl, this chapter is for you. We'll show you an organized, systematic approach to both tasks that will make them much easier and a lot more enjoyable.

The Plusses of Planning

We'll be the first to admit it: Meal planning and shopping aren't activities that rank high on the fun meter. Because of this, most people tend to not be as mindful about these tasks as they need to be. Instead of scheduling time for planning our meals and shopping for their ingredients, we often tack this time onto schedules that are already jam-packed with other activities. When the shelves in the refrigerator and pantry start to develop gaping holes, we go to the store for a marathon shopping spree that can easily last for hours. Or we zip into convenience stores to pick up items on the fly until we can make time for serious grocery shopping.

> **Dawn Says**
>
> With lifestyles the way they are today, we often run out of food before we make the next trip to the store. This lack of planning leads to more frequent trips to the vending machines and a greater reliance on fast food and convenience items. These items tend to be higher in calories and fat. They are also highly processed and lower in nutrients.

Both approaches are incredibly inefficient. Here's why:

♦ You'll spend more time in the store looking for items you think you need.

♦ You'll come home without some things that you need, necessitating a return trip.

♦ If you buy too much food, it will expire or go bad before you get around to eating it.

♦ You'll end up spending considerably more on your groceries than you need to.

Time is money when it comes to today's lifestyles. We can't afford to waste either of them. The good news is that you can quit spending more than you should on meal planning and shopping if you make some time for them on a regular basis. By regular, we mean sitting down and planning your meals weekly, and shopping for them weekly. That's it. Or if you're really pressed for time and you really hate to cook, you can hire someone to do your shopping and cooking for you. There are even services that will deliver meals to your home. They're expensive, but they're worth it for some people.

Most of us can't afford to turn our shopping and cooking over to someone else, so we're it when it comes to performing these tasks. If you've never planned your meals and you've never hit the grocery store with a list in your hands, getting your habits turned around will take a lot of work, especially in the beginning. As you keep doing it, however, it gets easier. Before long, you'll be a master shopper. What's more, you'll see results from your efforts. You'll …

- Spend less time at the store.

- Spend less money on groceries.

- Be less frustrated when you don't have the ingredients for certain meals on hand.

- Eat better because you have more healthy food choices on hand to pick from.

> **Eat It Up!** _____
>
> According to the Institute of Consumer Financial Education, the average American makes two trips a week to the grocery store and stops at a drug or discount store at least once a week. Even so, the NPD Group, an international marketing information company, reports that the time we spend on chores such as grocery shopping and meal preparation decreased during the 1990s. Time spent preparing food dropped 10 percent as home meal replacement and timesaving appliances became more popular. Grocery shopping time dropped 5 percent.

Marshaling Your Resources

There are a number of ways to organize meal planning and shopping. Most people take the old-fashioned approach: They determine what meals they're going to make over a certain period of time—say, a week—and they put together a list of ingredients for these meals.

Other people use store circulars for menu planning. Whatever is on sale during the week largely determines the meals they'll make. For example, let's say your local store is having a sale on whole organic roasting chickens. You decide to buy two—one for roasting this week, the other to freeze for later. Roast chicken will be the main entrée one night. Any leftovers can be used in sandwiches later in the week. Or maybe you can use them in that chicken tortilla soup recipe you cut out a couple of months ago—the ingredients for which you already have on hand.

> **Eat It Up!** _____
>
> If you want to get really fancy with menu planning, check out any of the software programs that are available for this. Many come with databases of recipes to choose from. They'll even analyze the recipes for their ingredients, and come up with a master shopping list for you to follow.

The key to success in menu planning is to find the system that works for you. Some families like to plan their weekly menus together. Other families find it easier to have one person be in charge of everything having to do with food preparation—planning, shopping, and cooking.

If that person is you, then you have your work cut out for you, but you'll also have more control over the process.

Regardless of the approach you take, you'll find that things will go more smoothly if you get organized before you start.

Recipes

If you use recipes when you cook, you probably have tons of them that you've clipped from newspapers and magazines that you haven't gotten to yet. If this is the case, take some time to sort them out. Sort them into three piles: The ones you want to try right away, the ones you'd like to try someday, and the ones you thought you'd use when you first clipped them but now have no idea why you did. Keep the first batch out. Put them to use by choosing one new recipe per week from the pile. File the second batch away, even if all you're doing is sticking them in a file folder for now. Toss the rest.

Coupons

The same thing goes if you're a coupon clipper. Go through all of your coupons and organize them into categories. If you don't have a coupon organizer, you may want to get one. They really make this task easier. Throw away any coupons that have expired. Pull out the ones that are ready to expire for your next shopping trip.

Foodstuffs

Sorting out the food you have on hand can take some time, so try to set aside a couple of hours where you can do it start to finish with as few interruptions as possible. Here's what you do:

1. Get out a yellow legal pad or other large note pad. You'll also need a trash can and a bag—the larger the better.

2. Go through every item on every shelf in your cupboards or pantry. Check the condition and expiration date of each. If you find any suspicious-looking packaging, or any items that are way past their expiration date, toss them in the garbage. It's usually okay to use packaged foods past their expiration date if they're not too old. Their quality might have degraded some, but they're usually safe. If you have food items that are more than a year past their expiration dates, however, then they should go. If you come across any items you don't think your family will use, put them in the bag for donation to a food shelf or shelter.

3. Take some notes on what you find as you go. For example, if you're long on canned tomato products, write down how much you have so you won't keep buying them. If you're low on items that you consider necessities, things like tuna fish, canned beans, and so on, note this as well.

4. If it's been a while since you've wiped down your shelves, do so as you're going through them. Wait until they're dry before you restock them. As you do, organize the food into categories. Group the cans of vegetables and fish together. Dedicate one shelf to pasta and other dry goods. Doing so will help you keep better track of what you have on hand. If you have items that are nearing their expiration dates, move them forward on the shelves so you reach for them first.

5. When you're done with your pantry, move on to the refrigerator and freezer. The process is basically the same. Here, however, you'll want to toss any food that is past its due date as these dates are more important when it comes to perishable foods. Also throw away anything that looks suspicious, even if it hasn't expired. Again, reorganize and clean the shelves and drawers as you go. Make notes on any basic food items that you're lacking and items you have an abundance of and need to use up.

When you're done with all of this, you'll have clean and well-organized food storage areas. You'll also have a good idea of what you have on hand and what you need to buy.

Some people even go so far as to make lists of the basic foodstuffs they want to have on hand. They then post these lists inside their cabinets or somewhere else in their kitchens. When the supply of a foodstuff is deleted, all they have to do is note it on the list.

> **Dawn Says**
>
> It's a good idea to clean and organize your kitchen on a regular basis—at least every two to three months. Doing so will help you keep on top of your food planning needs. It will also keep you from getting frustrated over not being able to find things.

Beginning with the Basics

Every kitchen needs to have basic supplies on hand. While individual needs vary greatly, there are certain items that virtually everyone has to have for basic food preparation. The list here was specifically developed to reflect the needs of active individuals and families. Some items need no refrigeration and have long shelf lives, so you can stock them to your heart's desire. Others need to be kept in the refrigerator at all times or after opening. Still others must be frozen. You can use this list to determine your basic kitchen needs. Add or delete items as necessary.

- Unsweetened baker's chocolate or cocoa. Buy the best you can afford. Carob powder is a possible substitute.

- Baking soda and powder

- Bouillon cubes or granules (choose low-sodium)

- Bread crumbs

- Canned and dried beans

- Canned or jarred peppers, both hot and mild

- Canned chicken, beef, and vegetable broth (low-fat, low-sodium, if possible)

- Canned fruit (water-packed or light syrup-packed only)

- Canned mushrooms

- Canned and dried soup

- Canned tuna (Other meats and fish, too, if you like them. Canned clams are great to have on hand to make clam sauce for pasta.)

- Canned vegetables

- Cereal, both ready-to-eat and ready-to-cook. Choose products that have minimal amounts of refined sugar and that are high in fiber.

- Chips and pretzels. Low-fat, low-salt are the best choices.

- Cooking oil. Best choices are canola oil and olive oil. Buy the best you can afford.

- Cornmeal (if you're buying organic cornmeal, you'll need to refrigerate it to keep it from going rancid)

- Cornstarch

- Crackers (low-fat, low-sodium)

- Evaporated milk

- Flour (again, if you're buying organic, it will keep best in the refrigerator or freezer)

- Frozen fruit

- Frozen vegetables

- Gelatin and pudding mixes

- Herbs, spices, and extracts. Whatever you need for cooking. If you keep the original containers you buy your herbs and spices in, you can refill them with bulk products for huge savings.

- Honey or another nonsugar sweetener

- Juice boxes or cans—both fruit and vegetable

- Ketchup and mustard

- Margarine and mayonnaise. Choose products that don't contain trans-fatty acids. Mayonnaise should be low-fat.

- Nonstick cooking spray

- Nuts. Best choices are walnuts, pecans, and almonds. The oil in nuts can make them go rancid fairly quickly. Store them in the refrigerator or freezer.

- Pancake mix. Find one made from whole grains.

- Pasta. Buy a variety of different kinds. Whole wheat is best, but it may take some getting used to and not all stores stock it. If you're buying regular pasta, select products made from semolina wheat as they're higher in protein. Stay away from products made from eggs if high cholesterol is a concern.

- Ready-made pasta sauces. Choose low-fat, low-salt, low-sugar varieties.

- Rice. Brown rice is best. Have a couple of other types on hand for variety. Jasmine rice is great with stir fry.

- Salsa. Choose low-salt varieties. Check the label closely for sugar. Believe it or not, some companies add it.

- Soy milk. Some varieties of soy milk are vacuum packed and have a shelf life of about a year. If it's not refrigerated in the store, you can put it in your pantry. Once you open it, you'll have to refrigerate it.

- Soy sauce

- Tofu. As is the case with soy milk, some tofu is vacuum packed and can last for a year or so on the shelf, but will need refrigeration when you open it.

- Tomato paste. Choose low-sodium brands.

- Tomato sauce. Choose low-sodium brands.

- Vinegar. It's a good idea to have a variety of different vinegars on hand as they're great flavor enhancers and they contain virtually no calories. Possible choices include rice vinegar (plain and flavored), tarragon vinegar, red wine vinegar, balsamic vinegar, and apple-cider vinegar.

- Wine (for cooking and drinking, if you so choose)

- Whole grains such as bulgur, buckwheat, barley, couscous, oatmeal, quinoa, grits, wheat germ, kamut, millet, and amaranth.

- Worcestershire sauce

With these basic items on hand, you'll never be stuck for a meal. You'll also be able to whip up appetizers in a moment when last-minute guests drop by. Here are just a few of the things you can serve using items from your pantry:

- Chips and dip. You can mash up canned beans and salsa for a quick party dip. Be sure to rinse the beans to remove as much sodium as possible before mashing.

- Spaghetti with white clam sauce.

- Baked tofu with spinach and tomato sauce.

- Crackers topped with tuna and jalapeno peppers (or mild red peppers if you prefer).

Having a good supply of basic foods on hand can go a long way toward making you feel like you're in control of your diet, instead of the other way around. Add a few perishables to this list—fruits, vegetables, dairy products, and so on—and you'll have a well-stocked kitchen that is up to making just about any meal imaginable.

Wise Sizing

When you're first stocking your pantry, you may be tempted to buy as much of everything as you possibly can so you don't run out in a hurry. Here's why this isn't a good idea: You don't yet know how much of anything you'll be using. That 64-ounce jug of cooking oil may look like a great bargain, but it's not if it turns rancid before you've used it up. The same thing goes for spices and other somewhat perishable shelf goods.

Eat It Up!

When you're stocking your pantry, make sure to buy food storage supplies such as plastic and aluminum wrap, waxed paper, storage bags, and plastic containers.

Even the most highly processed white flour will start to taste a little off if it sits on the shelf too long. Unless you can store these items in a cool place to keep them from spoiling or turning rancid, think small. Buy only as much as you think you'll use in a reasonable period of time, say three to six months. Or co-op your purchases. Find a friend or two with whom you can split the products and their cost.

Planning and Purchasing

Now that you have an idea of what your basic pantry needs are, it's time to put together a shopping list. Every household has certain foods that are used on a regular basis and need to be replenished often. These items will vary significantly, and no two households are alike in what they need to have on hand. If you're not sure what your household basics are, keep track of them for a week or two. Chances are your list will look something like this:

- Bread

- Cereal

- Fresh fruit

- Fresh vegetables

- Dairy products—milk, eggs, cottage cheese, yogurt, cheese, etc.

- Meat products—low-fat cuts of beef, chicken, turkey, etc.

- Snack items—things like juice boxes, granola bars, pudding cups, and other things that your family regularly grabs when hunger hits.

These items will form the basis for your weekly shopping list.

Next, add items to the list that you need for preparing specific meals. Dig out your recipes and your weekly planner. Figure out which meals you're going to eat at home and what they're going to be. Then choose some recipes to match.

Menu planning can be tough to do if you have an active family and especially so if there are specific dietary needs that must be met. Talk to your family and get their input on what they'd like to see on the menu. If you don't know what their schedules are, ask for this information, too. Then chart it all out on your planner. Or you can use the form in this chapter. When you have all of your information together, it should look something like this (due to space limitations, we're only showing you what a plan would look like for a few days):

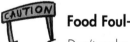

Food Foul-Ups

Don't make your menu plan too rigid. Build in some flexibility for things like last-minute practices or games that run overtime. If life is particularly hectic, don't choose dishes that take hours to prepare. Keep things simple.

	Sunday	Monday	Tuesday
Breakfast	buckwheat pancakes	cereal	leftover burritos
Lunch	tuna sandwiches	bag lunch	bag lunch
Dinner	pasta	burritos	game night (dinner with team after the game)

When you're all done, you'll have a list that includes the following:

◆ Pantry items (to restock supplies)

◆ Basics (things you need to buy every week)

◆ Extras (special items required for certain recipes)

To make things easier when you hit the store, you might want to sort your items into the following categories:

◆ Perishables, such as vegetables, fruits, dairy, bread, and protein items

◆ Nonperishables, such as canned foods and frozen foods

◆ Condiments

◆ Snack foods

Another way to sort your list is by how items are arranged in the grocery store. Many stores make available aisle-by-aisle lists for this purpose. Or you can simply walk the aisles of the stores you shop at to get a feeling for where everything is. What you'll find is that all grocery stores are pretty much arranged the same way. Perishables are on the perimeter; nonperishables are in the center. You'll find snack items and other impulse buys in the center of the store, on the ends of the aisle displays, and at checkout.

	Sunday	Monday	Tuesday	Wednesday	Thursday	Friday	Saturday
Breakfast							
Lunch							
Dinner							

Understanding the Playing Field

If it seems like supermarkets are set up to entice you into buying food that you didn't want, you're right. Food merchandising is a fine art, and food merchandisers spend millions analyzing consumer buying habits. They know exactly how to lure you and they know how to tempt you even before you set foot in a store. Nothing is left to chance when it comes to how shelves are stocked and what items are carried. Stores are even laid out in patterns that will keep you in them longer so that you'll buy more.

You can avoid many food merchandising traps by doing the following:

◆ Set a specific time limit for your shopping trip. If you go into the store planning to spend an hour, you won't waste time looking at items you have no intention of buying.

◆ Stick to the periphery of the store as much as possible. When you have to go into the center of the store, which is where merchandisers concentrate their efforts, figure out which aisles you need to shop, and shop only those aisles. Don't walk up and down every one of them. Some research says that as much as 85 percent of purchasing decisions are made while a consumer is looking at a product. If you don't look, you won't buy.

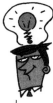

Eat It Up!

Feeling overwhelmed by all the choices in the grocery store? Small surprise there. According to the Food Marketing Institute, the average grocery store stocks more than 30,000 items. Every store has a different assortment of merchandise, which can boggle your mind even more if you shop at more than one store.

◆ Avoid impulse purchases by sticking to your list.

◆ Shop alone. This can be difficult if you have small children, but it is much more efficient. Plus, you won't have to deal with in-store tantrums when you refuse to buy your toddler the box of animal crackers that he or she can't live without.

◆ Get used to stooping and stretching. Food merchandisers fight over eye-level shelf space, and this is where you'll be barraged with special offers and premium food selections. Generic and lower-priced items are usually placed lower or higher on the shelves, rather than in the middle.

◆ Never shop when you're hungry. You'll be more likely to fall victim to special offers that wouldn't have as much appeal, or any at all, if your stomach wasn't growling.

Making the Rounds

The following is an aisle-by-aisle strategy to help you plan your shopping. All stores differ a little in exactly what foods they stock, but you should be able to find most of the suggestions here in any supermarket.

As previously mentioned, it's a good idea to spend the majority of your shopping time on the periphery of the store. This is where you'll generally find your produce, dairy, meat, and bakery sections. It's also where you'll be the least enticed by advertising and promotional gimmicks.

Wise Produce Buys

Pick a wide variety of fruits and vegetables. Fill your cart with color. If you're not naturally very adventuresome when it comes to these foods, try something new each week. Dark green, deep yellow, and orange-colored vegetables are generally highest in nutrients per serving. Select items that feel firm to the touch and that have minimal bruising. Avoid anything that looks or smells like it's seen better days—it probably has. If time is a concern, buy precut produce and lettuce in bags. It's more expensive, but the expense can be worth it. Keep perishable fruits and vegetables cool by selecting them toward the end of your shopping trip.

Banking on Bread

Look for bread products—including crackers, tortillas, pitas, and waffles—that list whole grains first on their ingredient lists. Choose products that are high in fiber and low in fat—3 grams or less per serving. For variety, try flat breads, lavosh, matzoh, bread sticks, bagels, English muffins, rice cakes, Melba toast, saltines, and whole-grain wafers.

Dealing with Dairy

Low-fat and no-fat choices are your best bet here. Be aware that many low-fat yogurts contain high levels of sugar. Check the label before you buy. You'll find soy products mixed with milk products in many dairy cases. Make your selections from this area toward the end of your shopping spree to minimize spoiling.

Meeting Up with Meat

Again, pick cuts that are as low in fat as possible. Be careful when buying ground turkey or chicken—it can contain skin and fat. Wrap these items in plastic bags before you put them in your cart to keep juices from dripping on other food items, and pack them separately from other items at checkout. In general, it's a good idea to avoid processed meat products—luncheon meat, bacon, sausage, etc.—as much as possible, as it's all high in sodium. Some bacon products are now available with reduced sodium.

Cashing In on Cereal

Cereal shopping (and the other categories that follow) will require moving to the center of the store. While here, look for cold and hot whole-grain cereals. You can tell whether they're whole grain if the grain is listed first on the label. Choose cereals that are low in refined sugar—less than 5 grams per serving—and high in fiber—at least 3 grams per serving or more.

Great Grains, Pasta, and Rice

Again, look for products that are high in fiber, such as whole-wheat pasta, brown rice, and whole grains. Avoid rice and pasta mixes as most are high in fat and sodium.

Scoping Out Snacks

Depending on the store, you should be able to find some healthy varieties of things like trail mixes, potato chips, tortilla chips, cookies, and so on. Look for low-fat products. Plain old popcorn is available everywhere. If you buy microwave popcorn, choose low-fat or no-fat products.

Banking On Beverages

When buying juice, choose items that are labeled 100 percent juice. Stay away from anything labeled as fruit beverage, punch, cocktail, or drink, as these products are mostly sugar water and contain very little real fruit juice. Carbonated beverages are tough to avoid buying if you like the taste of them. If you're trying to cut down on your consumption of them, try performance drinks or artificially sweetened flavored sparkling water.

Finagling Frozen Foods

Make these products your last choice before checkout. If you pack them into your cart next to meat and dairy products, it will help them all stay cold. Frozen fruit and vegetables are just as nutritious as fresh, so stock up on these items. Avoid vegetables that are packed with sauce and fruit that is packed in syrup. Many supermarkets now carry vegetarian entrées and other healthy products in their freezer sections. Other products you'll find here are flash-frozen, skinless chicken breasts, frozen fish, and soy burgers.

Money-Saving Strategies

Eating healthily comes at a price. Food that is higher up on the nutritional scale simply costs more. Soy products in general are more expensive than their nonsoy equivalents, but many people feel that the nutritional boost they get from eating them is well worth the additional cost. Organic fruits and vegetables are also more expensive, but they, too, are worth spending money on.

Some of the foods that athletes rely on to help fuel their performance are also expensive. Power drinks cost more than soft drinks. Good-quality whole-wheat bread is pricier than the white stuff. Those little juice boxes that your kids love to stick in their backpacks can make a big dent in your wallet. If you eat animal protein, you'll notice that lean cuts are more expensive. It can all get pretty pricey.

However, there are ways to reduce your overall grocery bill to lessen the hit from these foods. The following suggestions are just some of the things you can do to keep healthy eating from breaking the bank:

- ◆ Buy food in bulk whenever possible. Instead of purchasing individual boxes or bags of raisins, pretzels, chips, crackers, cereal, etc., buy large boxes, and divide the contents into small snack bags.

- ◆ Buy fruit and vegetables in season. Out-of-season items are always pricier.

- ◆ Use coupons as much as possible. If you're already a coupon clipper, you know the value in doing so. However, you aren't limited to the coupons you find in the paper or at the store. There are a number of Internet sites that also offer food coupons. You'll find some of them listed in Appendix B.

- ◆ Monitor your family's intake of perishable foods. If you're finding spoiled food in your fridge on a regular basis, buy smaller sizes more frequently so that they don't go bad before your family gets the chance to eat them.

- ◆ Store foods correctly to cut down on spoilage. If you need a refresher on this, check your refrigerator's usage guide, if you have it. County extension offices are another great source of information.

- ◆ Use food-saver bags to store fruits and vegetables. These handy products are a little expensive, but they do help extend the life of perishable goods.

- Buy generics and store brands whenever possible.

- Watch store ads for the best deals. Get to know the sales cycles at the stores you frequent so you can stock up on things at the best prices.

- Always check the reduced merchandise cart for day-old products and other marked-down items.

- If you have the space, stockpile nonperishable sale products.

- Watch unit pricing. Larger items often seem like a great bargain, but they aren't always cheaper.

- Shop at large chains whenever possible. Their greater buying power often translates into lower prices.

- If there's a food co-op in your area, consider joining it. Many co-ops sell bulk food in bins so that you can buy exactly the quantity you want. Less packaging also equals lower prices.

The Least You Need to Know

- Having nutritious food on hand at all times is the best way to keep healthy eating on track.

- Making menu planning and shopping a part of your regular routine will cut down the amount of time you spend doing both.

- Never shop on an empty stomach. Doing so is guaranteed to land unwanted food items in your cart.

- Avoid food merchandising ploys by sticking to your shopping list.

- Food that is high in nutritional value is often more expensive than less-nutritive items. You can minimize the hit on your budget that they make by shopping wisely, buying in bulk, and searching out the best deals.

Chapter 13

Bars, Gels, and Other Power Boosters

In This Chapter

◆ Boosting your energy with convenience carbohydrates

◆ Making the best bar choices

◆ Getting to know gels

◆ The benefits of sports drinks

While it's best to get your energy from food, more and more athletes are relying on energy gels, energy bars, and sports drinks to boost their carbohydrate stores and ensure maximum energy during long workouts and when they compete. If your activities last more than an hour or you're looking for an easy and convenient pre-workout snack, it's hard to beat these energy-providing powerhouses.

The World of Convenience Carbohydrates

Energy bars, gels, and sports drinks all provide on-call, on-the-go carbohydrate energy. They're easy to use and convenient, which makes them extremely popular. While they're all expensive sources of calories, there's no denying that they're about the most convenient way to boost your energy. They don't crush or spoil, and they're sold virtually everywhere. And there's no preparation time involved. All you have to do to fuel up is unwrap, uncap, or tear off a corner.

Which products are best for fueling your performance and keeping your energy levels high? It's pretty much up to personal choice. Gels are more concentrated than liquids and many people find them easier to digest than bars. Bars contain more calories than gels and sports drinks, but they can be hard to digest and they take longer to absorb. Both bars and gels require water to aid their digestion. Sports drinks tend to be the favorite since they're simple, quick, and easy. They taste good and you're getting carbohydrates and energy when you drink them.

Eat It Up!

Several studies have looked at the effectiveness of solid and gel carbohydrates versus liquid carbohydrates. The results: None have a decided edge over the other, but solid carbohydrates do need a water chaser to be most effective.

When choosing these products, be prepared to do some experimenting. They all vary widely in how they taste, and you'll definitely find some more to your liking than others. Some products are definitely more "tummy-friendly" than others, a factor that also varies widely. The bar, drink, or gel that your training partner loves might be great for him or her, but you might find them revolting.

Sports Bars

Sports or energy bars are so popular today that it's hard to believe they're a relatively new invention, only dating back some 20 years or so. Originally designed as an easily digestible, high-calorie, high-carbohydrate food for replenishing carbohydrate stores during long competitions, they're a favorite energy booster regardless of time or place. They're so widely available that many people eat them in place of candy bars. And, to be honest, there isn't much of a difference between the two when it comes to the calorie count and fat content of some of these products.

Eat It Up!

The first energy bar—the Power Bar—was invented in 1983 by Canadian marathoner Brian Maxwell as a way for athletes to replenish energy during races.

There are hundreds of different sports bars available in three basic formulations:

- High-carbohydrate, low-protein, and low-fat
- Balanced carb, protein, fat
- High-protein, low-carb

As the following chart shows, the calorie counts for sports bars can vary significantly, with the majority of them ranging between 200 and 300 calories. Their other contents also vary a great deal, which makes it important to read labels and pay attention to nutrient claims when choosing them.

Sports Bar Choices

Bar	Calories	Carbs	Fat	Protein (in grams)
Balance, Complete Nutritional Food Bar, Yogurt Honey Peanut	200	22	6	14
Balance Gold Crunch	210	23	6	15
Balance Outdoor, Honey Almond	200	21	6	15
Bear Valley, Fruit 'n Nut	420	59	13	17
BUT Stoker	252	48	3	10
Boulder Bar	210	40	3	8
Carbo-Crunch	180	60	19	20
Clif Bar	240	43	4	10
EAS Myoplex Deluxe, Chocolate	240	43	7	24
EAS Myoplex Lite, Toffee Crunch	190	28	3.5	15
Ensure Nutrition and Energy Bar, Cookies 'n' Cream	230	35	6	9
Edgebar	220	42	9	>2
Extreme Bar	230	44	3	7
Luna	180	24	4.5	10
Nature's Best Solid Protein Bar	290	8	7	30
MET-Rx BIG 100 Extreme Vanilla	330	53	1	27

continues

Sports Bar Choices   (continued)

Bar	Calories	Carbs	Fat	Protein (in grams)
MET-Rx Protein Plus	250	13	8	34
PowerBar, High Performance Energy Bar, Peanut Butter	230	45	2.5	10
Power Harvest, Apple	240	45	4	7
PowerBar Pria, Double Chocolate Cookie	110	16	3	5
PR Bar, Bavarian Mint	190	21	6	13
Thunder Bar, Chocolate	230	44	1	10
Tiger Sport, Vanilla	200	43	2	10
VO2 Max	230	45	3	5

Sports bars typically contain whey or soy protein as their protein sources (the soy-based products are sometimes marketed to women as a source of soy isoflavones). Those marked "outdoor" generally aren't chocolate covered and should hold up better when exposed to heat and other abuse, such as being smashed in backpacks or squeezed into pockets.

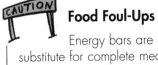

Food Foul-Ups

Energy bars are not a substitute for complete meals, even though some people use them as such. Regardless of what claims you might see on their labels, avoid using them as meal replacements if at all possible.

Best Energy Bar Choices

With so many bars available, trying to pick the right one can make your head spin. Rather than recommend specific brands, let's take a look at what you should look for when you're choosing one. If you want an energy bar to eat either right before or during an endurance event or long workout, choose one that is high in carbohydrates and low in fat and protein, which can hamper the absorption of the carbohydrates and cause stomach upsets. Bars that are high in carbs are great for providing glucose to working muscles and the brain for events or workouts that exceed 90 minutes.

Bars usually aren't necessary to fuel shorter workouts. For recovery, pick a bar that contains a minimum of .3 grams of carbohydrates per pound of body weight, plus at least 6 grams of protein and 0 to 30 percent healthy fat.

Regardless of the bar you choose, it's best to eat it well before you start working out in order to give the carbs it contains ample time to hit your bloodstream. About 30 to 45 minutes is optimal. And be sure to drink your water—anywhere from 8 to 16 ounces—while you're chewing away. If you feel sluggish during your activity, nibble on half of a bar every 15 to 20 minutes or so. And, again, don't forget to drink some water when you do.

Dawn Says
Don't wait until the day of an event or an important workout to test drive a new convenience carb product. Even liquid carbs can cause stomach upsets and hamper your performance. Experiment with all of these products at other times to determine which ones work best for you.

Energy Gels

Also called carbo gels, these are thick, smooth syrups or pastes that contain a mixture of simple and complex carbohydates. They come as small packets of plastic or foil with a tear-off end that makes it pretty easy to suck or gulp the contents out and get a speedy energy boost when you're on the move.

Energy gels provide more calories per ounce than sports drinks, and are easier to digest than bars. These handy pick-me-ups are available in tons of different flavors ranging from banana to vanilla. They also contain varying amounts of other ingredients such as vitamins, electrolytes, branch-chain amino acids, herbs, and caffeine.

 Eat It Up!

How do gels rate as an energy booster? One study conducted at California State University compared gels to placebos. Although researchers didn't measure performance, they did report higher levels of blood glucose (sugar) in the athletes who consumed the gel when compared to the placebo group. This indicates that using gels when exercising will spare carbohydrates stored in the muscles and extend endurance.

Energy gels provide between 70 to 120 calories and 17 to 30 grams of carbohydrate per packet. Because they're fat free, they'll leave your stomach quickly and hit your bloodstream fast.

Product Name	Calories	Carbohydrates	Caffeine
Carb-Boom	107	27 g	Vanilla Orange contains caffeine
Clif Shot	100	24 g	Mocha Mocha and Sonic Energy Gel Strawberry contain the equivalent of $\frac{1}{2}$ cup of coffee
GU Energy Gel	100	25 g	All flavors except Banana Blitz contain caffeine (the equivalent of $\frac{1}{5}$ cup)
HammerGel	100	23	Espresso contains caffeine
Power Bar PowerGel	110	28	Chocolate contains 25 mg of caffeine; Tangerine contains 50 mg.
Honey Stinger Natural Energy Gel	112	28	Ginseng has caffeine

Since there is no protein, fat, or fiber in sport gels, they are rapidly absorbed into the bloodstream. Each pack provides enough carbohydrate to fuel about 30 minutes of energy.

As with bars, choosing a gel is pretty much an individual preference. Unlike bars, though, gels don't differ much when it comes to nutritional composition as they all contain about the same amount of carbohydrates and calories. If you want to use them, try several different brands to see which ones taste good to you. Consistencies do vary between brands, so you'll also want to find a product that appeals to you and sits well in your stomach. Many gels contain caffeine. Some studies suggest that it may improve performance by reducing fatigue during endurance activities; however, the amount you get in gels probably isn't enough to affect your performance either way. While caffeine has not been proven to be harmful in small amounts, it does affect many individuals

Dawn Says

Gels are liquid, but they're extremely thick liquid, which means that they're not a source of fluids. It's just as important to drink water when you down them as it is to chase your energy bars with H_2O. Taking several good gulps of water with each pack of gel will enhance their absorption.

adversely, so the benefits of using it must be weighed against its pitfalls. If you are trying to avoid it, be sure to choose gels that don't contain it.

Sports Drinks

The first sports drink, Gatorade, was developed by scientists at the University of Florida as a hydration aid for members of the school's football team. It's still the best-known sports drink out there, but there are many others to keep it company.

Today, sports drinks fall into three basic categories:

♦ Sport or electrolyte replacement drinks, which are designed to aid in hydration and contain low amounts of carbohydrates and sodium. Products in this category include Gatorade, the first commercially available carbohydrate-based "energy" product; Cytomax, Exceed, PowerAde, All Sport, and Hydra Fuel.

♦ Carbohydrate loading drinks, which, as their name implies, are used to help the body store more carbohydate prior to competition. These products contain more carbohydrate by volume than sport drinks do. Products in this category include GatorLode, Exceed High Carb, Ultra Fuel, Carbo Force, and Metabolol Endurance.

♦ Recovery drinks, which are designed to speed recovery following intense workouts or competition by refueling muscle glycogen. They also contain protein to help repair the muscles. Products here include NitroFuel, Power Surge, Pure Pro, and Mass Recovery.

Like bars and gels, there are tons of different sports drinks on the market. If you're going to use them, make sure you select the appropriate product for your needs. Sport or electrolyte replacement drinks are good if you're going to be exercising or competing for more than an hour at a fairly good exertion level. The best choices are those that contain high percentages of fast-absorbing carbohydates—glucose, sucrose, and glucose polymers or maltodextrins.

If you don't have problems with heat cramps, drinking a mixture of half water/half sports drink should meet your hydration needs. You'll need to take in anywhere from 16 to 32 ounces per hour depending on your size, exertion level, temperature and humidity conditions, and your regular rate of fluid loss. For the best results, start drinking before you start exercising and keep drinking them every 15 to 20 minutes or so, just like you would with water. If you do experience heat cramps, nix the water and guzzle the sports drink. The electrolytes will help prevent them.

Carbohydrate loading drinks are meant to be used prior to endurance competitions, although some individuals are now using them during events that last longer than four hours. If you do, you'll want to look for products that are low in fat as too much of it can hamper their absorption. Recovery drinks, of course, are meant to be used after working out or competing. For best results, drink them immediately after and up to two hours after exercise.

The Least You Need to Know

- Convenience carbohydrates can provide an extra energy boost for intense or long workouts.

- Your best-choice energy bars will be high in carbohydrates and low in fat and protein.

- If you plan to use bars or gels for fuel during an event, experiment with them well in advance to find the ones that work best for you.

- Sports drinks come in a variety of formulations that range from keeping you hydrated to helping you recover after a tough workout or a long competition. Be sure you choose the right product to meet your needs.

Chapter 14

Buying Supplements and Performance Enhancers

In This Chapter

- ◆ Defining dietary supplements
- ◆ Learning how to determine supplement quality
- ◆ Choosing the best antioxidants
- ◆ Hot and not-so-hot sports supplements

Somewhere along the line, it's bound to happen. You'll get aced out in a race by your training partner who you beat handily the year before. Or you'll see someone you know at the gym who was a spud a few months ago and is now cut and trim and looking like you wish you did. Ask them the secret behind their amazing transformations and they tell you either a little or a lot about some new supplement they're taking that's the next thing to a miracle cure.

It seems like everyone's searching for some sort of Holy Grail, a product that magically packs on muscle, decreases body fat, improves endurance, or helps us live longer. What's more, there are tons of companies fueling our quest by making products that just might do what we're looking for.

Walk into any store that specializes in these items and your head will spin with terms like amino acids, BCAAs, HMB, phytochemicals, beta carotene, lycopene, and so on. And what's with all those herbs? Is any of it worth the money?

Some of it is and some of it isn't. In this chapter, we'll give you the lowdown on the supplements that work, the ones that are dubious, and the ones you should stay away from. We'll also tell you how to read the labels so that you know what's in those bottles and what you need to know to buy the best.

Understanding the Dietary Supplement Industry

There's a certain amount of caveat emptor ("buyer beware") concerning the world of supplements and performance enhancers—dietary supplements, in legal terms. As you'll soon see, these products are regulated to a certain extent, but the scrutiny they receive is nothing compared to what prescription drugs are put through before they're approved. For this reason, just about anyone can manufacture and market a dietary supplement product as long as they follow the regulations. What they don't have to do, however, is prove that their products actually work.

Foodie

Dietary supplements are defined by law as products that contain one or more of the following dietary ingredients: a vitamin; a mineral; an herb or other botanical; an amino acid; a dietary substance used to supplement the diet by increasing the total daily intake, such as enzymes, organ or glandular tissue; a concentrate, metabolite, constituent, or extract; or a combination of these ingredients.

The main reason there are so many different dietary and herbal supplement products on the market today is that the industry isn't highly regulated. The Food and Drug Administration oversees dietary and herbal supplements, but its oversight is limited, for the most part, to how products are marketed. (The Federal Trade Commission also plays a role in regulating the supplement industry and oversees claims that are made in advertising and marketing materials.) When it comes to what these products actually contain and how they're manufactured, the burden of proof regarding safety and efficacy falls on the manufacturer, not on the government.

The FDA's role in regulating the supplement industry was established by the Dietary Supplement Health and Education Act passed by Congress in 1994. This act did the following:

- Defined dietary supplements and dietary ingredients

- Established new guidelines for assuring safety and for displaying literature where supplements are sold

- Established guidelines for statements and claims that could be made about nutritional supplements

- Required ingredient and nutritional labeling

- Gave the FDA authority for establishing good manufacturing practices, or GMPs, that would govern the preparation, packaging, and storage of dietary supplements

The law stopped short of giving the FDA direct authority for ensuring the quality, safety, and efficacy of these products. Unlike prescription drug manufacturers, supplement manufacturers do not have to prove that their products can deliver desired or specific benefits. However, they are responsible for ensuring that the products they make or distribute are safe, and that any claims or representations made about these products are not false or misleading.

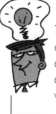

Eat It Up! _____

The Dietary Supplement Health and Education Act governs how vitamins, minerals, herbs, and specialty supplements are regulated by the federal government. It also affirms the importance of studying the relationship between supplements and disease prevention, and it helped establish the Office of Dietary Supplements within the National Institutes of Health to stimulate and support this research.

In addition, there is nothing in the DSHEA act requiring dietary supplement manufacturers to conform to specific manufacturing practices beyond those already established for foods, or for their products to contain specific formulations or ingredients. This means that the amount of active ingredients in a supplement could range from significant to miniscule. Because of this, a supplement manufactured by one company may be vastly different from another supplement that contains the same ingredients manufactured by someone else.

The FDA does regulate what supplement companies can and can't say on their labels. Manufacturers can't:

- Claim that their products prevent, cure, or treat any disease or ailment.

- Imply that the use of a supplement is a cure.

- Use a trademark that implies a cure.

Labels must provide information on the amount and weight of the different components in the supplement, the recommended serving size or usage instructions, and must mention all botanical and herbal ingredients. Herbal supplements must also identify the part of the plant used in the product. Labeling can also make claims related to the following:

- Nutrient content, such as stating that a product is high in calcium or vitamin C.

- Health benefits. Here, the FDA authorizes claims only where there is a documented relationship between the supplement and a disease or health-related concern, such as potassium reducing the risk of high blood pressure and stroke, or calcium lowering the risk of osteoporosis.

- The product's effect on the body's structure or function. A label for standardized horse chestnut, for example, can say that it "supports healthy circulation in the legs." A label for spirulina can say that it supports a healthy immune system, supports normal cholesterol levels, and boosts energy and cellular health. Products making these claims must also carry a disclaimer that reads, "These statements have not been evaluated by the FDA. This product is not intended to diagnose, treat, prevent, or cure any disease."

Dawn Says

The best supplement manufacturers adhere to a set of federal regulations called Current Good Manufacturing Practices (cGMPs), which were established by the FDA to ensure the safety and quality of food products. Another set of standards that are important to the supplement industry are those set by the U.S. Pharmacopeia (USP), which assure the potency, uniformity, disintegration, and dissolution of each product. When researching supplements, make sure the ones you choose are manufactured by companies that meet industry standards for good manufacturing practices and USP.

The FDA is also authorized to take action against any dietary supplement deemed to be adulterated or unsafe, including restricting product use or pulling products from the market. The FTC steps in when companies make claims above and beyond the ones stated here. It can make companies suspend advertising that makes false claims and sue violators. While some people believe that the government could have done more to protect the rights and health of consumers when it comes to dietary supplements, the DSHEA is actually a big step in the right direction. Before the bill was passed, there was no legislation that specifically addressed how dietary supplements should be regulated. The FDA made judgment calls on whether they were foods, drugs, or food additives, depending on their intended use, and regulated them based on the requirements they had established for these products. What the DSHEA did was to determine that dietary supplements should be regulated based on the same safety requirements that the FDA imposes on foods. This put the burden on the manufacturers to ensure that their products are safe and properly labeled.

What's on the Label

All dietary supplements must carry nutritional labeling. Similar to the Nutrition Facts label that food products must carry, the Supplement Facts label must include …

- Serving size.

- Servings per container.

- The amount per serving for each dietary ingredient or blend (the source of the ingredient may also be included, such as zinc from zinc citrate).

- The Percent Daily Value (DV), which details the percentage of the recommended daily intake for each nutrient that the supplement provides.

- A list of the ingredients that don't appear in the Supplement Facts information panel. These generally are the inert ingredients used to give the product its appearance or shape, as well as any preservatives that are used. These ingredients are listed by weight in descending order.

Nutritional labeling also must include the manufacturer's or distributor's name, address, and zip code. Finally, the terms "dietary supplement" or similar terms such as "herbal supplement" must appear somewhere on the product label as a general description of product.

Thanks to the DSHEA, we also know more about the role that dietary supplements play in disease prevention and health promotion than ever before. Remember the Office of Dietary Supplements? Since its establishment, the OCD has conducted or supported a number of studies, including ones that …

- Established safe upper limits for B-vitamin intake.

- Examined the role of antioxidants in preventing cataract development in people with diabetes.

Eat It Up!

Dietary supplements that contain macronutrients, like protein powders, must carry the same Nutrition Facts panel that other foods do.

- Studied the role of calcium supplements in reducing short-term changes in bone density in male and female high school students.

- Examined the actions of zinc and copper in proper brain development and function.

Even with a greater emphasis on dietary and herbal supplement research, we have only begun to scratch the surface on what we know about these products. In the years to come, you'll see much more information on the role they play in preventing disease and promoting good health, as well as more information on how they can be used.

Now that you know more about how supplements are regulated, let's take a closer look at how you can use this information to help you choose the supplements that will deliver the results you want.

Choosing Quality Vitamin and Mineral Supplements

Remember what we said earlier about no two supplements being alike when it came to their ingredients? Because there are no specific standards set for what these products can contain, their efficacy—that is, the results they can deliver—run the gamut from being highly effective to not doing much at all.

Vitamin and mineral supplements may look a lot alike when you see them on the shelf, but they can differ greatly when it comes to what they'll do for you. For this reason, it's not the best idea to saunter into a store and grab the first bottle of multivitamins you see. They might be a good product. Then again, they might not. The only way you'll be able to tell is by doing your research.

The product label will tell you some of what you need to know. From reading the label, you'll be able to tell the following:

- How much of each nutrient the product contains. The best ones will have at *least 100 percent* of the daily value established for each essential nutrient.

- If the supplement is an antioxidant formula, meaning that it contains higher levels of these nutrients.

- What form the nutrients are in, such as vitamin C as ascorbic acid or vitamin E as d-alpha tocopheryl succinate.

What the label can't tell you is how well you're going to absorb these nutrients. Everyone absorbs things a little differently, so a product that works great for you might not work as well for someone else. It also won't tell you if the form that the nutrients are in is the best. For example, vitamin E and carotenoids are best when they are in their natural form, because the body doesn't absorb synthetic forms as well.

Dawn Says

I highly recommend that everyone take a high-quality multivitamin/mineral supplement. Do your research in this area. Before jumping on the bandwagon for a particular product, look at the label and ask about the research that supports the claim. A solid nutritional company will be able to get you this information in a reasonable amount of time. Once you receive the information, make sure it is current and from a reputable journal. Evaluate how the study was done. If this seems too time-consuming, find a health professional—preferably a dietitian who specializes in sports nutrition—who knows about supplements, and find what might work for you.

The forms of antioxidant vitamins that appear later in this chapter are all higher up on the absorption ladder. Find them in the supplements you're considering and the chances are good that you're holding a quality product in your hand. If you are, you can expect to pay more for it, too. While cost isn't always an indication of quality in the supplement world, it is true that vitamins that contain better ingredients will be more expensive than those that don't.

Understanding Bioavailability

The amount of the supplements you take that your body absorbs—their bioavailability—is affected by a number of different factors, including the supplement itself—its form, when you take it, and how you take it. Other factors, such as consuming alcohol, smoking, eating poorly, having high stress levels, or taking certain prescription drugs, can also inhibit nutrient absorption.

Minerals, which aren't digestible in their natural form, need to be "chelated," or put through a process that binds them to an amino acid, which makes them more easily absorbed. Certain vitamins and minerals should be taken in combination with other nutrients to enhance their absorption. They include these:

◆ Vitamin A. It should be taken at the same time as you take other fat-soluble vitamins because they work better together. It's also good to chase vitamin A with food that contains fat, such as peanut butter, which binds with the nutrient and boosts absorption.

- Vitamin B. The B vitamins work best if they are taken as part of a B-complex formula.

- Vitamin C. Bioflavonoids—the chemicals that form the pigments in plants—enhance vitamin C absorption and retention. Quercetin, rutin, and hesperidin are the bioflavonoids found naturally with vitamin C. Grapeseed extract also boosts absorption.

- Vitamin E. Take with vitamin A for best synergistic benefits. Since vitamin E easily oxidizes in the body, it's best to take this vitamin in several small doses during the day instead of one megadose.

- Calcium. Vitamins C and D boost absorption of this important nutrient. Magnesium also works together with calcium. For best results, choose a supplement that combines calcium and magnesium in a 2:1 ratio.

If you take a multivitamin/multimineral supplement, you won't have to worry as much about getting the best combinations.

Synthetic vs. Natural Vitamins

Vitamins can be derived from natural sources or formulated in laboratories. In general, vitamins in their natural form are going to be more expensive than those that are made in a lab. However, the different forms that vitamins take aren't always an indication of how well they're going to work. There are a few vitamins, however, that you should always try to get in specific forms as they are more easily absorbed by the body. They are these:

- Vitamin C. Esterified C contains various forms of vitamin C that work synergistically.

- Vitamin D. The label should say cholecalciferol.

- Vitamin E. The natural form is d-alpha tocopherol. The synthetic version is dl-alpha tocopherol.

- Carotenoids. These are substances such as alpha and beta carotenes, lutein, lyopene, and zeaxanthins. Your body converts what it needs to vitamin A and uses the other carotenoids as antioxidants. If you're going to take these, buy only natural carotenoids.

Certain forms of minerals are also better absorbed than others. In general, those that are identified as citrates, chelates, or aspartates are better absorbed than sulfates.

One Pill vs. Many Pills

For ease of use, most people like to take a multivitamin supplement that contains all the vitamins and minerals they think they need in one tablet. This isn't a bad place to start, but many multivitamins don't contain everything you need. If you're going to take the "multi" approach, consider taking separate multivitamin and multimineral supplements. Your chances of getting the full complement of essential nutrients will be vastly improved.

The other problem in taking an "all in one" pill is that your body can't use all the vitamins it gets at once. The better approach is to take supplements at least twice or three times daily. An easy way to remember to take them is to time them with meals. Doing so not only boosts their absorption, it also helps the body metabolize other food components.

What should you look for in a good multivitamin/multimineral supplement? Experts say it's best to find supplements that are low in fillers and additives—the things that hold the tablets together. The supplements you take should also contain at least 100 percent of the daily value for the major nutrients and should be formulated whenever possible from forms of vitamins and minerals that are known to be ones that the body absorbs well.

You should see the following information on a good-quality supplement:

- A complete list of ingredients and amounts
- The form of each ingredient—e.g., calcium in the form of calcium citrate
- Full address of the company, not just a post office box number
- Expiration date
- A notation that the company follows Good Manufacturing Practices (GMP)
- Third-party certification proving manufacturing quality
- A notation that more information, including research, is available by contacting the manufacturer

Getting the Right Antioxidants

Many people are tossing aside their basic multivitamin/multimineral formulations for supplements that contain higher levels of the nutrients that have antioxidant properties and that contain other substances, such as bioflavanoids, which also function as antioxidants. Since there are many different kinds of free radicals, which means that no single antioxidant will wipe them all out, this makes a lot of sense.

For optimal cell nutrition, it's important to take higher doses of vitamins and minerals with antioxidant properties than of other micronutrients. Doing so will give your body the best defense against degenerative diseases. The following chart lists the main categories of antioxidants, their best forms, and their recommended daily values. As noted, with some antioxidants you'll want a mix of the different forms, because your body will use them better. Others are simply available in various forms and sometimes a mixture of these forms is better.

Antioxidant	Form	Amount
Vitamins		
Vitamin A	Beta-carotene	10,000–15,000 IU
	Alpha carotene	500–800 mcg
	Lutein/Zeaxanthin	1–6 mg
	Lycopene*	1–3 mg
Vitamin C	Calcium, Potassium, Magnesium, and Zinc Ascorbates	1000–2000 mg
Vitamin D	Cholecalciferol	450–800 IU
Vitamin E	d-alpha tocopherol, d-gamma tocopherol, mixed tocotrienol	400–800 IU
Vitamin K	Phylloquinone	50–100 mcg
Alpha-Lipolic Acid	Alpha-Lipolic Acid	13–30 mg
Vitamin B1	Thiamin HCL	20–30 mg
Vitamin B2	Riboflavin	25–50 mg
Vitamin B3	Niacin and Niacinamide	30–75 mg
Vitamin B5	Pantothenic Acid as D-Calcium Pantothenate	80–200 mg
Vitamin B6	Pyridoxine	25–50 mg
Vitamin B12	Cyanocobalamin	100–250 mcg
Biotin		300–1000 mcg
Folate	Folic Acid	800–1000 mcg

Antioxidant	Form	Amount
	Bioflavanoids	
Bilberry		Amounts vary
Broccoli		Amounts vary
Bromelain		Amounts vary
Grapeseed Extract		30–90 mg
Green Tea		Amounts vary
Quercetin		Amounts vary
Rutin		Amounts vary
	Minerals	
Calcium	Calcium Citrate, Calcium Carbonate	800–1500 mg
Chromium	Polynicotinate, Picolinate	200–300 mg
Copper	Copper Gluconate	1–3 mg
Iodine	Potassium Iodine	100–200 mcg
Magnesium	Magnesium Citrate, Amino Acid Chelate, and Oxide	500–800 mg
Manganese	Manganese Gluconate	3–6 mg
Molybdenum	Molybdenum Citrate	50–100 mcg
Vanadium	Vanadyl Sulfate	30–100 mcg
Zinc	Zinc Citrate	20–30 mg
	Other Nutrients	
CoQ10		12–30 mg
Glutathione		10–20 mg
Choline	Choline Bitartrate	100–200 mg
Inositol		150–250 mg
Olivol	Olive Extract	30 mg

It's best to take a mixed carotenoid containing all of these substances. Your body will convert what it needs of the alpha and beta carotenes to vitamin A and use the other carotenoids as antioxidants.

All About Performance Enhancers

When it comes to looking for a product that will deliver the competitive edge, performance enhancers lead the list. They fall into a variety of different categories, with the following being the most common:

- ♦ Workout boosters that provide energy to muscles

- ♦ Products that rev up metabolism and help burn fat, including carnitine and creatine

- ♦ Substances that support muscle growth and performance, such as amino acids, vitamins, and herbals

- ♦ Recovery enhancers, such as drinks that contain carbohydates and electrolytes or protein

Food Foul-Ups

Performance enhancers are not a substitute for a good diet. Eating right is always going to be the best way to ensure optimal performance. And don't look to these products to be overnight miracles. With most of them, it can take a while—sometimes months—before you feel their effects.

There are tons of different products available, which make selection difficult. What makes it even more difficult to choose a performance enhancer is the fact that they don't work the same for everyone. An energy booster for one person might not have an effect on another.

Before taking any performance enhancer, take a close look at what you're eating and see if you need to make any adjustments there to meet your specific goals. If not, buy small amounts of anything you're going to try. Give it a few weeks to see if it's working. Stop taking any product immediately if you experience negative side effects.

Hot Performance Enhancers

Here are some of the most popular performance enhancers that have been shown to have some beneficial effects:

Beta-hydroxy beta-methylbutyrate (HMB). This is a metabolite of the amino acid leucine. It may help minimize protein breakdown during intense exercise, leading to less muscle damage and improved muscle mass and strength. Research supports its ability to improve lean tissue and strength when paired with resistance training. Dosage: 3 to 5 grams/day during heavy training.

Branch Chain Amino Acids (BCAAs). BCAAs are three of the essential amino acids—isoleucine, leucine, and valine—that comprise muscle protein. These three amino acids account for about 35 percent of the amino acid content in muscle tissue. Supplements are believed to stave off fatigue, increase endurance, improve energy levels, and improve mental performance. They might be of value for athletes participating in endurance sports, such as road cycling, triathlons, and marathons. As BCAAs may also decrease muscle breakdown following exercise, they're also popular with bodybuilders. Dosage: 5 to 20 grams per day.

Choline. Choline is a B-vitamin that plays a role in brain development and muscle contraction. It is believed to help promote energy and delay fatigue. In one study, 7 out of 10 marathon runners who took choline before competing improved their running times by more than five minutes. Dosage: 600 to 1,200 mg/day.

Chromium. One of the more popular supplements on the market today, chromium is a trace mineral that is believed to help the body burn fat while building muscle. It also plays a role in glucose metabolism. While deficiencies are rare, too little chromium results in insulin resistance. Some studies suggest that chromium supplementation can improve the body's ability to break down and use carbohydrates during activity. Most people don't get enough chromium through what they eat, and supplementation has shown to be effective in maintaining proper insulin function and helping some dieters lose weight. Dosage: 50 to 200 mcg per day.

CoQ-10, or Coenzyme Q-10. CoQ-10 is an enzyme that can be found in all cells. It helps to convert food, oxygen, and water into energy. It also acts as an antioxidant that helps prevent cell damage from free radicals produced during strenuous exercise. Athletes use it as an energy booster; however, research doesn't support its use in this arena. Dosage: 100 to 200 mg/day.

Creatine. One of the hottest of the hot supplements, creatine is an amino acid that the kidneys and the liver naturally synthesizes from arginine, glycine, and methionine. It's been studied in depth, unlike many other dietary supplements, which means we know a great deal about how it works. Research shows that it can improve performance during highly anaerobic activities such as sprinting, diving, jumping, and weightlifting as it increases production of phosphocreatine, which is needed for the phosphagen energy system. However, there is nothing to support its benefits for endurance athletes. One study found that female athletes who consumed creatine over a five-week period experienced a substantial gain in weight-training strength compared with those who were given placebo. Dosage: loading dose of 20 to 25 grams per day for 5 to 10 days, and then 2 to 5 grams a day as a maintenance dose. Usually taken with a high-carbohydrate drink, like fruit juice, to aid absorption.

Glutamine. Another amino acid that is found in the body, glutamine plays a role in the synthesis of other amino acids and glucose. Glutamine is also important to immune functioning and plays a role in cellular replication. Research supports using glutamine to maintain muscle mass and support immune system function. It is also believed to help counteract the catabolic, or muscle-wasting, effects of stress hormones such as cortisol, which can be elevated by strenuous exercise. Dosage: 1 to 20 grams per day during periods of heavy muscular exertion.

Glycerol. Glycerol is a liquid alcohol that is a component of triglycerides or fat. It helps the body store water, and some athletes use it to boost their water stores before endurance competitions. Bodybuilders like it because it helps muscle cells retain water and increases muscle definition. Dosage: 1 gram per kilogram (2.2 lbs) of bodyweight taken in about 6 to 8 ounces of water or sports drink, beginning about 90 minutes before activity starts.

L-Carnitine. L-Carnitine is another amino acid that is synthesized in the liver and kidneys from lysine and methionine. It plays a role in the metabolism and transfer of fatty acids into the mitochondria of the cells for energy production. Research supports its use as an energy aid as it boosts fatty acid metabolism, thereby lessening the body's dependence on carbohydrates for energy. Dosage: 250 to 500 mg per day for regular use; during intense training 2 to 4 grams per day.

Methyl-sulfonyl-methane (MSM). MSM is a natural sulfur compound that is found in the body and in a variety of foods, including green vegetables, meats, seafood, tea, coffee, and milk. It is used to reduce pain, soreness, and inflammation caused by injuries or overuse. While there is little scientific evidence to support these claims, one study showed that athletes who used MSM had less pain and soreness after hard training. Dosage: 250 to 750 mg per day.

NADH (nicotinamide adenine dinucleotide). NADH is a coenzyme that plays a role in energy production. It stimulates ATP production, which can help raise energy levels and reduce fatigue. It also helps transform the amino acid tyrosine into dopamine, an important brain chemical. Dosage: 2.5 mg daily as a maintenance dose, or 10 to 15 mg taken at least 1 hour prior to activity.

Phosphatidylserine (PS). PS is a phospholipid—a fat-soluble substance that is an essential component of cell membranes. It is essential for healthy cell function, especially in the brain, where it is found in high concentrations. Studies have shown that PS can help reduce cortisol levels, and therefore decrease soreness and muscle damage. It might help athletes recovering from long, strenuous activity such as marathons. Dosage: 1,000 to 2000 mg immediately before or after intense training.

Pyruvate. Pyruvate is a carbohydrate that results from glucose metabolism. It is purported to help burn fat, increase lean muscle mass, and increase endurance. Studies suggest that it may be helpful in preventing weight regain after loss. Dosage: 3 to 15 grams per day.

Ribose. Ribose is a simple sugar found in all the cells of the body. It forms the carbohydrate portion of ATP, DNA, and RNA. Ribose helps fuel strength and endurance performance. Studies have shown that it helps improve anaerobic performance and restore ATP levels after short-burst, high-intensity exercise. Dosage: 3 to 10 grams per day.

Whey Protein. Derived from milk, whey protein is one of the most popular protein supplements on the market today, and for good reason: It is easy to digest, rich in BCAAs, and low in fat. Studies show that it boosts immune level functioning. It also enhances the production of glutathione, a powerful antioxidant. Whey protein is very popular among bodybuilders and other athletes who want to gain muscle mass but can't get enough protein in their regular diet to support their efforts. Dosages vary.

Not-So-Hot Performance Enhancers

These products either have little data to back up their claims or can be downright dangerous to take:

Androstenedione. This is a precursor, or prehormone, of the male sex hormone testosterone. It's reputed to boost lean muscle mass and enhance performance, although more than several studies have disputed this. It can also raise levels of estrogen in men, which could lead to enlarged breasts. Dosage: Androstenedione should not be taken by women of any age, or by men under age 21. For men over 21, no more than 300 mg per day.

Ephedra (ma huang). Used in traditional Chinese medicine for thousands of years to treat certain respiratory symptoms, ma huang contains ephedrine, which is a nervous system stimulant. It creates heat by speeding up the body's metabolism, which leads to its wide use as a fat burner. It can also boost energy. Taken in too high of a dose, or when combined with other stimulants, it can cause the jitters, insomnia, high blood pressure, seizures, and even heart palpitations, heart attacks, strokes, and death. Dosage: no more than 8 mg of ephedrine (the active ingredient) at a time; no more than a total of 25 mg in one day.

The Least You Need to Know

- The Food and Drug Administration oversees the dietary and herbal supplement industry.

- Supplements and performance enhancers are regulated to a certain extent, but manufacturers don't have to prove that their products actually work.

- Vitamins can be derived from natural sources or formulated in laboratories. In general, vitamins in their natural form are more expensive than those that are made in a lab.

- Performance enhancers have different effects on different people. Buy small amounts of any products you're going to use until you know that they work for you.

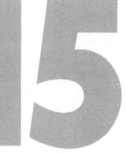

Nutrition on the Go

In This Chapter

- ◆ Best fast-food choices
- ◆ Avoiding fast-food pitfalls
- ◆ Best nutritional traveling companions
- ◆ Avoiding the vending machine blues

Is your schedule in control of you? Or are you in control of your schedule? If the first statement is the better description of what your life is all about, your good nutrition could be going right out the window.

Busy lifestyles and hectic schedules can turn a balanced diet into a nutritional nightmare, especially if you eat a number of your meals on the run. It is possible to eat healthily and well when you are on the go, but it usually takes some advance planning to do it right.

Fast-Food Society

We have definitely turned into a society that eats on the run more often than not. According to researchers, nearly one in six dinners is eaten somewhere other than around the dining room or kitchen table.

According to the 1994–1996 Continuing Survey of Food Intakes by Individuals, a greater percentage of Americans are eating away from home than ever before. In 1994 and 1995 (the most recent years available), 57 percent of Americans ate at least one food away from home on any given day, up one third from 1977–1978 when 43 percent of Americans ate away from home.

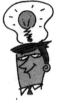

Eat It Up!

Researchers say that teenage boys are most likely to eat away from home, with almost three quarters of them obtaining and eating at least one food outside of the house on any given day. Individuals over age 60 are least likely to eat away from home.

From Cafe to Car Seat

Decades ago, eating out generally meant sitting down to a meal in a restaurant, cafe, diner, or maybe at a lunch counter. Every so often Mom and Pop might give the kiddies a special treat and take them to a drive-in for a hot dog or a burger with fries on the side. But those days are long gone. Today, eating out is more about grabbing a handful of food on the fly when we're rushing from one place to another. We're still sitting down to our meals, but we're doing it behind a steering wheel.

Unlike previous generations that considered going out to eat something of a special occasion, eating out has become a way to fit meals into a much-too-busy life. Here are some more statistics on outside-the-home eating habits, just to give you a better idea of what's going on:

- ◆ Our favorite eating-out spots are fast-food restaurants.

- ◆ Just over a quarter of the people who eat out choose a restaurant with table service.

- ◆ About one quarter of the people who eat out buy and eat food from a grocery or convenience store without ever bringing it into the house.

- ◆ The meals most often eaten away are lunch or brunch, followed by a snack or beverage snack.

- ◆ About a quarter of individuals eat their breakfasts away from home on a regular basis.

Our love of eating out is great news for the fast-food and convenience store industries, but it isn't doing much for our health. While it is possible to eat healthily when eating on the go, many people use their hectic schedules as an excuse for indulging in "Just this one time won't hurt" thinking and they make food choices that are anything but good for them. Doing so occasionally isn't that big of a deal. Having a bacon cheeseburger, cola drink, and fries at your favorite fast-food stop isn't in itself a diet-buster, especially if you show some self-constraint and don't "super-size it."

The key word here, however, is occasional. When your favorite fast-food combo meal becomes the fall-back lunch or dinner more often than not, it can wreak havoc in two places: your wallet and your waistline.

> ### Dawn Says
>
> If you just can't live without an occasional fast-food burger or burrito, build them into your eating plan so you can enjoy them as treats every so often and not feel like you're being deprived.

The High Cost of Eating Away from Home

Eating out is considerably more expensive than eating at home or eating meals that you've prepared at home and brought with you. The sandwich or piece of fruit that you grab at a convenience store can cost two to three times more than a similar item that you slap together on your kitchen counter or pluck out of your refrigerator. Not only that, but they can be considerably lower in nutritional value. Prepackaged sandwiches and other quick meals like hot dogs, burritos, and so on can also be high in saturated fat, preservatives, and salt.

The same goes for fast food. It, too, is considerably more expensive than eating at home, and it can come at a huge cost to your health. Many fast-food choices are laden with saturated fat—a known contributor to atherosclerosis and coronary heart disease. A good number of them also contain high-fructose corn syrup, which has been linked to rising obesity rates, because the body processes this sweetener differently than it does sucrose or dextrose. Many fast-food items are also high in calories. A typical fast-food burger meal can provide between 50 and 75 percent of the recommended daily calorie intake for most individuals. When that meal comes on top of normal calorie intake, it pushes calorie levels above where they should be. The result is weight gain, especially if the additional calories are not offset by increased physical activity.

While it's true that fast food can be a nutritional nightmare, it's important to put things into perspective when it comes to exactly what this nightmare is. Regular fast-food items—burgers, fries, shakes, and so on—are always going to be higher in calories, fat, sugar, and sodium than food found virtually anywhere else. However, an even bigger

 Eat It Up!

The smallest bag of french fries at McDonald's contains 210 calories for 2.4 ounces of fries. Supersize those fries and the calorie count jumps to a whopping 610 calories for 7.0 ounces.

problem with fast food these days is portion size. The difference between 4 and 10 Chicken McNuggets is 300 calories. A McDonald's cheeseburger is 330 calories. Substitute a Quarter Pounder with Cheese Deluxe for that cheeseburger, and the calorie count jumps up to 530.

The same thing is true when it comes to that home delivery favorite—pizza. Again, pizza is always going to be relatively high in fat and sodium—that's a given. Eating a few pieces of a medium pepperoni pizza, however, isn't going to break your nutritional bank if you don't do it that often. But most people don't order a medium pizza. Large and extra-large are the favorite take-out and home-delivery sizes. Not only will the nutritional counts be different between slices of medium and large pizzas, but you'll also probably eat more when you order a large, simply because it's there.

While healthy is still a relative term in the fast-food arena, it is possible to find alternatives to high-fat, high-sugar, and high-calorie offerings on almost all fast-food menus. We'll talk about how to do it later in this chapter. Even the occasional home-delivery pizza or take-out Chinese dinner can be part of a well-balanced diet.

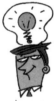

Eat It Up!

Wondering what the nutritional values are for your favorite fast food? Do an Internet search on the company name. All the major chains now provide this information on their corporate websites.

Fast-food companies and convenience stores are not the only places offering unhealthy food choices. You are going to be confronted with them everywhere you go. You can avoid putting your eating plan into free fall by knowing which foods to choose when you eat away from home. You can also avoid it by planning ahead so you can minimize your reliance on drive-up windows, vending machines, and convenience store coolers.

Mapping Your Strategy

Reducing your reliance on fast food can be one of the best things you can do for your nutritional health. It might not be easy—especially if you're used to letting your schedule control your life—but if you stick to it you can be successful.

A good way to start is by mapping out your schedule for one week. Get a yellow pad or a calendar and list all of your activities for each day. (If you don't keep an appointment calendar on a regular basis, you'll want to start doing so.) A sample day might look something like this:

6 A.M. Get up

6:15 A.M. Morning bike ride

7 A.M. Shower

7:45 A.M. Put Joey on bus; catch shuttle to office

10 A.M. Meeting with client to discuss merger (away from office)

11:30 A.M. Lunch

1 P.M. Finance group meeting

2:30 P.M. Conference call with headquarters

4 P.M. Meet with Kim to review presentation

5 P.M. Catch shuttle to rec. center; watch Joey in soccer practice

5:45 P.M. Collect Joey and friends; meet Sue for dinner

7 P.M. Supervise homework

8 P.M. Work on presentation for tomorrow

9 P.M. Wipe out! Long day; time for bed

This is a fairly typical schedule. It might look a lot like one of yours. It gets a B for detail, but an F for good nutrition. Take a closer look at it and you'll notice the following:

1. It doesn't include breakfast. Given a typical morning for most people, if breakfast isn't entirely skipped, it's probably being eaten on the fly, possibly as a fast-food muffin or breakfast burrito.

2. It doesn't include a preworkout snack. Again, this isn't to say that there isn't one, but it's not on the schedule.

3. It includes two meals eaten away from home. Although we don't know for sure, at least one meal is probably at a sit-down or fast-food restaurant.

4. There are no scheduled midmorning or afternoon snack breaks. If food is being eaten at these times, selections are probably coming out of a vending machine.

The following schedule reflects healthy food choices made as the result of some advance planning:

6 A.M. Get up

6:05 A.M. Preworkout snack of $1/2$ slice whole-wheat bread topped with a tablespoon of natural peanut butter. Put out cereal box, juice, and milk for Joey.

6:15 A.M. Run—let's see if I can go a little faster this time.

7 A.M. Shower

7:45 A.M. Put Joey on bus with lunch packed the night before. Take shuttle to work. Buy container of fat-free milk from street vendor to put on cereal stored in desk.

8 A.M. Eat breakfast. Chase cereal with milk and juice (also from box stored in desk).

9:45 A.M. Midmorning snack selected from fridge stash.

11:30 A.M. Lunch out with Bob from purchasing. He likes to eat healthily— no problem here.

1 P.M. Planning committee meeting.

2:30 P.M. Afternoon snack, again selected from fridge or desk stash.

5 P.M. Catch shuttle to rec center to watch Joey play soccer.

5:45 P.M. Dinner with Sue. The kids want burgers; we'll choose a place close to home that has dinner salads for the adults.

6:45 P.M. Walk home from restaurant.

7 P.M. Supervise homework while making breakfast and lunch for tomorrow— it's an eat-in day at work.

7:45 P.M. Walk the dog.

8 P.M. Put together grocery shopping list for the weekend. Work on presentation.

9 P.M. Bedtime.

A schedule like this borders on overkill, and it probably has more detail in it than yours ever would, but it makes several important points. With some advance planning, and some thought put toward making good food choices, a hectic schedule can also be a healthy one. It can also include some additional exercise, which is always a good thing.

Not planning ahead is one of the top reasons why we depend so heavily on fast food, vending machines, and other unhealthy food options. Spend a few minutes on a food plan and you won't be a slave to convenience foods.

The second schedule also illustrates some great strategies for healthy eating on the run. Let's take a closer look at some of them.

> **Dawn Says**
>
> The best plans take into consideration the needs of all family members. It's not always possible to gather everyone around and ask them what's on their agendas for the week, but the more you know about their needs, the easier it will be for you to plan ahead for them.

Breakfast on the Go

According to researchers at The HPD Group, more Americans are eating breakfast on the run than ever before. On-the-go and skipped meals accounted for 21 percent of all breakfasts in 1999, compared to 17 percent in the early 90s.

Although we don't often think of breakfast as a meal that can be packed ahead of time, this is just one strategy for eating it away from home. If you like cereal, for example, then toss a serving into a snack-sized plastic bag and munch on it as you're going to work. You can wash it down with milk at the same time or have a milk chaser when you get to the office.

Other on-the-go breakfast strategies include the following:

- Keeping breakfast bars, packaged dried fruit, and low-fat crackers in your car or desk at the office. Match them up with milk, yogurt, low-fat cottage cheese, whole-wheat bagels, or fruit, either from home or purchased at a convenience store.

> **Dawn Says**
>
> Always have breakfast. This is the one meal of the day that you can't afford to miss.

- Stock up on easy-to-carry breakfast foods at home that have long shelf lives, such as dried fruit, breakfast or snack bars, low-fat crackers, fruit or vegetable drinks, cereal cups, and ready-to-eat cereal. Nonrefrigerated pudding snacks and gelatin snacks are also good choices. Keep them together in a special place in your pantry so that you always know how much you have on hand.

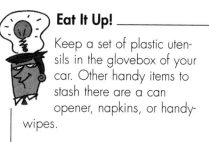

> **Eat It Up!**
>
> Keep a set of plastic utensils in the glovebox of your car. Other handy items to stash there are a can opener, napkins, or handy-wipes.

- Cook in bulk. Make enough cooked cereal or egg dishes to last for a few days. Split them into individual servings and refrigerate or freeze. In the morning, either pop them into the microwave at home or take them to work and cook them there.

Lots of people skip breakfast because they aren't hungry in the morning. If you're one of them, start with fluids like juice or milk. Save solid food for later in the morning when your appetite kicks in.

Savvy Snacking

The same think-ahead philosophy applies to midmorning and afternoon snacks. Unless there are vending machines with healthy food choices where you work, you'll need to plan ahead to avoid the call of the doughnut tray when hunger pangs strike.

Dawn Says
Keep your internal engine stoked at all times by eating something every three to four hours. Even fast-food or less-healthy options are better than nothing at all. If you go too long without food, you'll eat more when you finally get the chance to eat and the calories you take in may very well surpass that of the fast-food snack.

Stashing your food in your desk or refrigerator at work is the best way to make sure that you have healthy snacks on hand. Easy-keeping foods include these:

- Dried fruit
- Trail mix
- Energy bars
- Unsweetened cereal
- Low-fat crackers and chips
- Plain popcorn
- Pretzels
- Canned tuna
- Low-fat or no-fat pudding cups
- Soy nuts
- Premixed protein shakes
- Artificially sweetened gelatin snacks
- Canned fruit

If you have access to a refrigerator, stock up on things like low-fat or nonfat yogurt, string cheese, soy milk, fresh fruit, raw vegetables, and juices.

Noontime Nutrition

If you didn't like carrying your lunch to school, packing a bag meal to work might be the height of dorkiness to you. However, it's just about the best thing you can do for your budget and your waistline. Even eating cheaply doesn't get you away from the food counter without spending at least a few dollars. Substitute that lunch-counter lunch with one from home and you can easily save at least $10 to $20 a week. Do it for a year and you could have enough money saved for a great vacation or that snazzy trail bike you've had your eye on for a while.

Bag lunches can go far beyond the classic combo—sandwich, chips, carrot sticks, apple, and cookie. Try some of the following lunches for a new twist on the old standby:

- Cup of soup and low-fat crackers. Low-fat bean-based or lentil soups are good choices here.

- Chicken or baked tofu wrapped in lettuce leaves. Pack some olive oil or tahini to drizzle on top for an extra treat for your tastebuds.

- Hummus (chickpea spread) on whole-wheat crackers or pita

- String cheese and a whole-wheat bagel

- Tuna in a can with whole-wheat pita bread

- Peanut butter with low-fat whole-wheat crackers

Add fresh veggies and either water-packed or fresh fruit to each selection for a complete meal.

Digging In When Dining Out

If eating in restaurants is a big part of your life, it's important for you to get savvy about making good food choices wherever you go. Fortunately, there aren't many restaurants that are off-limits when it comes to eating out if you know what to look for and you're assertive about your needs. In fact, it's possible to eat healthily at even the greasiest greasy spoon.

Some restaurants are just naturally better nutritional choices than others. Oriental restaurants are top picks because Far Eastern cuisine emphasizes fresh vegetables and low-fat protein choices like fish and tofu. Seafood restaurants are another obvious choice, as are places that specialize in vegetarian cuisine.

Food Foul-Ups _____

Avoid restaurants with menus that say "no substitutes." These establishments often buy prepared food—such as fish or chicken coated in batter or breading, or vegetables that are already swimming in butter or cheese sauce—that has to be cooked in a certain way. While you can pick the batter or breading off or pick the veggies out of their fat-laden surroundings, better choices are restaurants that prepare their food in a healthier manner to begin with.

Decoding the Menu

As previously mentioned, you can find healthy food choices at almost any restaurant. If you see any of the following terms on the menu, you're in good shape:

- Broiled
- Steamed
- Char-broiled
- Grilled
- Boiled
- Poached
- Marinara
- Tomato sauce
- Au jus (in its own juice)

These are all low-fat preparation methods. You won't go wrong with any of them.

Avoid selections that have the following terms in their descriptions:

- Fried
- Pan-fried
- Battered
- Batter-dipped
- Crispy
- Breaded
- Scampi-style

- Creamed or cream-style

- Buttery or butter-flavored

- Au gratin

- Gravy

While these preparation methods can add lots of flavor to food, they also add lots of fat. If you're interested in a dish that has any of these descriptions associated with it, ask if an alternative preparation style is possible—for example, if vegetables could be served plain instead of creamed or au gratin. Grilling is often an option for pan-fried fish.

There are lots of little dietary traps just waiting to trip you up when you eat out. The rice pilaf that comes along with your healthy chicken breast entrée might have been cooked with butter. Salads might be pretossed with dressing. If you aren't sure about how something will come, ask. You might not be able to change the way the food is prepared, but you might be able to make a healthier substitute. If you're a vegetarian or a vegan, you'll have to be especially careful. Many seemingly innocent entrées—even pasta—might contain animal protein.

Ordering off the menu—in other words, asking for a special dish of your own devising that doesn't appear on the menu—is another option for when you're dining out, especially at better restaurants that put a premium on pleasing their customers. It never hurts to ask. Some chefs actually welcome the opportunity to prepare healthy dishes for customers who ask them to do so. The worst you'll hear is "Sorry, we can't."

Food Foul-Ups

Not only are we eating larger portion sizes when we dine out, we're doing it at home as well. Researchers from the University of North Carolina at Chapel Hill have found that food portion sizes in restaurants and at home have increased over the past 20 years. While pizza portions decreased, portions of salty snacks increased from 1 ounce to 1.6 ounces, soft drinks increased from 13.1 fluid ounces to 19.9 fluid ounces, hamburgers increased from 5.7 ounces to 7 ounces, french fries increased from 3.1 ounces to 3.6 ounces, and Mexican food increased from 6.3 ounces to 8 ounces. Fast-food establishments serve the largest portion sizes; restaurants serve the smallest portion sizes.

Managing Portion Sizes

It's also important to keep an eye on how much food you're served when you eat out. Portion sizes in most restaurants are huge—some places serve up dishes so big that they can feed two people.

Some restaurants will allow two people to split one entrée (sometimes at a slight additional cost), or will serve reduced portion sizes if you ask for them. If not, you'll have to get creative. Use your portion-sizing skills to figure out how much you can eat. If you're served a baked potato that's as big as both your fists put together, eat half and leave the rest. Pasta can be harder to eyeball, but not impossible. A good starting point is to simply cut the portion you're served in half. If it still looks like more than a cup or so of noodles, halve it again.

What should you do with your leftover food? Taking it home in a doggie bag is an obvious answer. If you're too embarrassed to ask for one, you can ask your server to pack up your food for you.

Ordering à la Carte

At many restaurants, meal prices include soup or salad, vegetable, and some sort of starchy carbohydrate along with the entrée. Other restaurants offer their menu items à la carte, meaning that each item is priced separately. Dining in these establishments tends to be more expensive, but such pricing can give you more ordering flexibility as well. Instead of getting a complete dinner with all the fixings, you can choose exactly what fixings you want.

> **Dawn Says**
>
> You can keep things under control when eating at a buffet by making salad your first course. Stay away from anything other than plain greens and dress them with oil and vinegar, not one of the calorie-laden dressings that grace most buffet tables. After you're done eating your salad, go back for your entrée.

Avoiding Buffet Busts

All-you-can-eat extravaganzas can be great bargains, but often they're only great for your pocketbook. Buffets are dangerous when it comes to portion control. They aren't nicknamed "troughs" for nothing.

If you must eat at a buffet, do it wisely. Survey the food tables before loading up your plate. Target the most nutritious-looking choices and take only what you want of them. If some less-healthy items are beckoning you, just take a dab of each.

Healthier Fast Food

Although most fast food is higher in fat, sodium, and sugar than what you'd eat in other places, you can still find healthy food choices at almost any outlet. Your best bet is to eat at fast-food spots that post the nutritional information for the foods they serve or that make this information available if you ask for it. Some chains have even put together healthy menu choices to guide you.

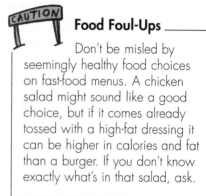

Food Foul-Ups

Don't be misled by seemingly healthy food choices on fast-food menus. A chicken salad might sound like a good choice, but if it comes already tossed with a high-fat dressing it can be higher in calories and fat than a burger. If you don't know exactly what's in that salad, ask.

Basic strategies for fast-food eating include:

◆ No "supersizing." Stick to regular-sized portions to keep things under control. If there's a kiddie menu, consider ordering off it.

◆ Staying away from breaded or fried foods. Look for dishes described as grilled or char-broiled.

◆ Ordering items you know to be good nutritional choices, such as plain chicken-breast sandwiches, plain baked potatoes, and salads. Keep them good choices by avoiding high-fat dressings and other condiments. Replace mayonnaise-type sauces with mustard, ketchup, or salsa.

◆ Making wise choices when it comes to dairy products. Shakes are often made with ice milk, which is low in fat, but this doesn't mean that they aren't high in sugar. Frozen yogurt might be low-fat. Then again, it might not be. If you're not sure, ask. If the information isn't available, stick to low-fat or nonfat milk.

Always remember that some of the healthier choices found on many fast-food menus are healthier only when compared to the other items on those menus. Others are nutritional stars. McDonald's, for example, offers five different salads ranging in calorie counts from 35 to 150 (before dressing). Top them with fat-free or low-fat dressing, and you've got a darn good lunch going.

Eating Right When You're on the Road

You can even keep your good nutritional habits going when you're traveling. Again, think ahead and be prepared. If you regularly travel by air, you already know that many airlines have drastically reduced or even eliminated their in-flight meals. Know what to expect by calling ahead. If your flight includes food service, ask if you can order a special meal. If food service is provided, low-fat, low-sodium, low-calorie, or vegetarian meals are often available. The best time to make this request is when you book your flight. It's a good idea to confirm your special request 48 hours before you fly.

If your flight doesn't include meal service, or if it includes something that you know you won't want, pack a meal to take with you. Your best choices will be from home, but many airports also offer healthy foods that you can grab on the run if you're pressed for time.

Many hotels and motels offer rooms with refrigerators and microwaves. You may have to pay more for them in some places, but you can't beat the convenience of having them. Find a grocery store or supermarket and stock your mini-kitchen with water, veggies, fruit, and other healthy items.

If you're traveling by car, avoid having to eat at truck stops and fast-food chains by packing meals for your trip.

The Least You Need to Know

♦ Having limited time doesn't mean you don't have a choice of what you put in your body.

♦ Keeping your nutritional program on track calls for planning ahead whenever you need to eat away from home.

♦ Fast food isn't off-limits when eating out. Do your homework and know what your choices are before you start ordering.

♦ You can keep late-afternoon or evening bingeing under control by taking along a healthy snack for eating between meals when you're on the go.

Chapter 16

Eating Before and After Competition

In This Chapter

- ◆ Best pregame foods
- ◆ Proteins vs. carbohydrates
- ◆ Recipes for before the game
- ◆ Recipes for after the game

By now you've heard the gospel often enough that you should know it by memory, but we'll repeat it one more time: Eating the right foods, and eating them at the right times, can improve your performance no matter what sport you play or activity you participate in.

You now know all about the building blocks to good nutrition—the macronutrients and the micronutrients you need for preventing diseases and promoting good health. In this chapter, we put it all together for you and tell you what you need to eat and when. As a bonus, there are tons of great recipes on the pages ahead that will make eating right easier than you ever thought it could be. So, eat up!

General Guidelines

The food you eat before competition or working out has to contain enough carbohydrates to fuel your performance. This is especially important if you're going to be active first thing in the morning. When you're sleeping, your body loses some of its carbohydrate stores. This happens even if you're eating the way you should throughout the day.

Dawn Says

No matter what, make sure you eat something before you work out or compete in the morning, even if it's just a bite of something. Asking for optimal performance from your body when it's fasting is about the worst thing you can do to it. It rapidly depletes liver and muscle glycogen and will impair your performance.

The same thing is true for after-competition eating. You need foods that are high in carbohydrates after an activity in order to replenish your body's glycogen stores.

In planning your meals, keep the following considerations in mind:

◆ What you like to eat

◆ When you need to eat

◆ The digestibility of the foods you want to eat

Eat It Up!

The old training table diet of steak and eggs is definitely a thing of the past. Some athletes are so wedded to it that it fuels their minds more than their bodies, but meals like these that emphasize protein and fat over carbohydrates have been shown to hamper performance, not enhance it.

Down with Protein, Up with Carbs

In general, you'll want to emphasize carbohydrates and minimize foods that are high in protein and saturated fat the day before competition. These foods digest slowly and remain in your digestive tract longer than carbohydrate-based foods with similar energy contents.

As a reminder, here's why carbohydrates are the hands-down gold standard when it comes to pre- and postcompetition eating:

◆ They replenish glycogen stores in your liver and muscles that are lost when you're sleeping.

- Your body digests and absorbs them faster than proteins or fats, which means they'll provide energy faster. Plus, they won't make you feel weighed down after you eat them.

- They take less energy to metabolize than proteins and fats do. They also take less water, so the risk of getting dehydrated during competition is lower.

- Eating or drinking carbohydrates shortly after you finish working out or competing will make this vital macronutrient more available to your muscles at a time when they need it the most.

> **CAUTION**
>
> **Food Foul-Ups**
>
> Eating right before and after exercising or competing won't erase the damage done by less-than-optimal eating at other times. A healthy pregame meal might help your performance to a certain extent, but it won't have the same benefit as it would if you were taking in the right nutrients, and enough of them, on a regular basis.

Carbohydrates are simply the best energy source you could ask for. Stick to them when you're eating for performance, and you just won't go wrong.

When to Eat

When you eat is as important as what you eat. In general, three hours is sufficient time for digesting a carbohydrate-rich precompetition meal. If you don't have enough time to eat a full meal, eat a smaller meal or a snack that provides the same carb boost and is low in protein and fat.

If you tend to be on the jittery side before you compete, you probably already know that being nervous or edgy makes it difficult to find foods that don't upset your stomach. However, you still need to eat. To do so, you'll have to eat foods that you know you can digest well, which means you'll have to experiment with them well before event day. One possibility is a recovery drink (recovery drinks were discussed in Chapter 13). They contain carbohydrate to fuel performance, along with enough protein and fat to help you feel full.

Recovery drinks can also save the day during long events—marathons, tournaments, meets, and the like—where other kinds of food might be in short supply and there isn't much time to eat them anyway.

Watering Up

The importance of staying hydrated when you're active just can't be stressed enough. Make sure you take in enough fluids to keep you hydrated. If it's hot, you're going to need more than your usual 8 to 10 cups a day. Drink before, during, and after competition. If water doesn't appeal to you for some reason, sports drinks are an excellent option because you'll get carbohydrates and electrolytes along with your water.

Pregame or Training Meals

The following recipes form the basis for training meals that can be eaten three to four hours before an event. They are good sources of energy and they provide the right proportions of carbohydrates, protein, and fat. They're great for parent groups who cook for teams. Just copy the recipes and distribute them to the members of the group. We've also given you some suggestions for side items that will turn these dishes into complete meals.

One of the things you'll note is that these recipes emphasize the importance of getting your carbohydrates from a number of sources. Some people think that pre-event eating means chowing down on bowls full of pasta and not much else. While pasta is a good source of carbohydrate, it's a much better one when paired with other healthy carbs. Your best pre- and postgame eating, especially an hour or two before the event and right after it, depends less on starchy carbohydrates like pasta and beans and more on fruits and vegetables that are more easily digested.

If you're feeding small children with these menu plans, decrease the serving size of all foods equally. Don't just serve a normal size of the entrée and take out the side items. Follow the same rule if you need to increase serving sizes. Putting the food on the plates before you bring them to the table will keep portion sizes in better control. If you provide a choice of vegetables you'll increase your chances of their liking one of them. Serve a sports drink, 1 percent or skim milk, 100 percent fruit juice, or water.

Rita's "Cloned" Famous Restaurant Potato Soup

Serve with broccoli-carrot slaw tossed with low-fat or fat-free slaw dressing and salt-free crackers. This is good with skim milk as well.

1½ cups chopped onions

Buttery spray or 1 tsp. olive oil

4–6 cups diced potatoes with some skin left on if desired

2–3 cans, 14.5 oz. ea., fat-free, low-sodium chicken or vegetable broth

1½ cups half-and-half

½ cup nonfat dry milk powder

1½ cups dry instant mashed potato flakes (optional)

Salt and pepper to taste

Put onions in nonstick pan and spray with buttery spray or sauté in a teaspoon of olive oil. Cook for a few minutes and add potatoes. Stir. (You can use cooked potatoes or leftover baked potatoes, in which case your soup will be done in record time.) Add broth and bring to a boil. Boil, if using raw potatoes, until potatoes are tender, about 15 to 20 minutes. If using cooked potatoes, bring to a boil and lower to a simmer. Add cream and continue to simmer a few minutes. You can now purée some of the potatoes with a hand blender or mash with a potato masher, or leave as is and start adding potato flakes to thicken the mixture. Stir to blend and add seasonings to taste. Serves six to eight.

The recipe alone

Calories: 296

Carbohydrates: 61 percent 46g

Fiber: 4g

Protein: 17 percent 12g

Fat: 22 percent 7g

Saturated Fat: 4.5g

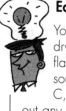

Eat It Up!

You can always add some dry, instant mashed potato flakes to thicken any cream soup for a boost of vitamin C, calcium, and iron without any added fat.

Note: If you want smoother soup, try Yukon Gold potatoes. Russet or baking potatoes have more starch, giving this soup a naturally thick base.

Easy Lasagna

This recipe can be divided in half or make the whole batch and freeze half. You can substitute four whites for the eggs or the equivalent of egg substitute.

2 containers fat-free ricotta cheese, 15 oz. ea.

2 large eggs

2 cups reduced fat mozzarella, shredded

1 cup fat-free Parmesan cheese, grated, or fat-free Parmesan blend

2 jars, approx. 28 oz. ea. chunky style garden pasta sauce (reserve 1 cup sauce) and then mix remaining sauce with 1 cup water

12 uncooked whole-wheat lasagna noodles

Combine ricotta, eggs, 1 cup mozzarella, and ½ cup Parmesan. Layer 4 uncooked noodles, 1 cup sauce and half of ricotta mixture; repeat. Top with 4 uncooked noodles and sauce. Cover with foil. Sprinkle with rest of cheeses and bake in preheated 375-degree oven for 1 hour. Remove foil and bake another 10 to 15 minutes. Let stand 10 minutes. Serve with reserved sauce, heated. Serves 12.

The recipe

Calories: 235

Carbohydrates: 42 percent 23g

Fiber: 4g

Protein: 34 percent 19g

Fat: 25 percent 6g

Saturated Fat: 2.5g

Serve with a salad of hearty mixed greens and fat-free Italian dressing, steamed green beans, skim or soy milk and Italian bread to up the energy and carb count. When you do, the overall percentage of protein in the meal will drop, making it optimal for a training table meal.

Pasta Parmesan

8 oz. low-fat or fat-free cream cheese

¾ cup skim milk

½ cup fat-free Parmesan cheese

1 clove garlic, minced

1 TB. light tub margarine (the kind that's 4.5 grams fat per serving/tablespoon)

8 oz. whole wheat or regular pasta, cooked

½ cup shredded carrots

2 cups fresh chopped greens or 1 cup blanched broccoli florets or other fresh vegetables, blanched (optional, but good)

Melt cream cheese and milk in nonstick pan. Add Parmesan, garlic, and margarine. Blend. Pour over hot pasta and toss with carrots and greens. Serves four.

Calories: 209

Carbohydrates: 52 percent 25g

Fiber: 2g

Protein: 35 percent 16g

Fat: 14 percent 3g

Saturated Fat: 1g

Add a glass of skim milk and a fruit cup with fat-free whipped cream. This will up the energy and carbs and decrease the protein percentage.

Pasta Puttanesca

1 TB. olive oil

2–3 tsp. garlic

1 lb. whole-wheat or regular pasta, cooked

$1/4$–1 tsp. red-pepper flakes

1–2 tsp. anchovy paste

1 can (28-oz.) low-sodium diced tomatoes

2 TB. capers (optional but good)

2 oz. chopped black or green olives

Add oil to skillet. Add garlic and cook for 1 minute. Add pepper, anchovy paste, tomatoes, and capers. Bring to a boil. Lower to simmer and cook about 10 minutes. Ladle over pasta. Serves four.

Option to up the protein and energy: Add 1 to 2 cups of red kidney beans to the recipe.

Calories: 250

Carbohydrates: 63 percent 40g

Fiber: 4g

Protein: 12 percent 8g

Fat: 25 percent 8g

Saturated Fat: 0g

For some people, 250 calories might not be enough. To up the energy needed for a training meal you can add more vegetables, fruit, or even a smoothie or fat-free ice cream for dessert.

Pasta Fagioli

This recipe can very easily be halved if necessary. Serve with a salad of mixed greens and French bread.

1 lb. whole-wheat or regular pasta, boiled

2 TB. olive oil

1 TB. minced garlic

1/2 tsp. red-pepper flakes

28 oz. canned diced tomatoes

1 1/2 to 2 tsp. oregano

2 cans beans, approx 15 oz. ea. cannelloni, chickpeas, kidney, or your choice, drained

1/2 lb. fresh spinach, torn or other greens such as chard, kale, etc.

Fat-free Parmesan blend for sprinkling on top

Heat oil, garlic, oregano, and red-pepper flakes over low heat until garlic smells fragrant but does not brown, about 2 minutes. Add everything else but spinach and Parmesan blend. Bring to a boil. Lower to a simmer and cook 10 to 15 minutes. Stir in spinach. Cook just until wilted. Pour over cooked pasta. Sprinkle with plenty of Parmesan blend. Enjoy!

Calories: 235

Carbohydrates: 70 percent 23g

Fiber: 4g

Protein: 18 percent 19g

Fat: 12 percent 6g

Saturated Fat: 2.5g

These percentages are great for a meal. This is also a great vegetarian option.

Cranberry Almond Biscotti

This great dessert is high in carbohydrates and has virtually no fat. It's easy to make, too. You can use any dried fruit you like—cherries, chopped apricots, raisins, etc.

2 cups flour

1 cup Splenda

1½ tsp. baking powder

1 cup dried cranberries

3 large eggs, room temperature

2 tsp. ea. vanilla and almond extract

Additional Splenda to sprinkle on top (optional)

Preheat oven to 350 degrees. Mix flour, Splenda, and baking powder in food processor or mixer. Whisk eggs and extracts in another bowl until beaten. Add egg mixture to flour mixture and process or mix until combined. Mixture will be somewhat sticky and thick.

Grease or spray a cookie sheet. Divide dough into two parts and transfer to cookie sheet. Shape into two 8" long, ½" high loaves. If desired, sprinkle with a small amount of Splenda.

Bake for 20 to 25 minutes until pale golden and center of loaf is firm when touched. Remove from cookie sheet and cool a few minutes. With serrated knife, slice each loaf on the diagonal into ½" slices. Cut each slice lengthwise into two and bake again 8 to 12 minutes or until desired crunchiness is reached. Or leave as is for a softer cookie. Store in covered container at room temperature. Makes 48.

Calories: 30

Carbohydrates: 88 percent 6g

Fiber: 0g

Protein: 11 percent 1g

Fat: 2 percent 0g

Saturated Fat: 0g

Southwestern Rice and Beans

Serve with salad made with three different greens and choice of fat-free dressing, French bread and skim or soy milk.

1 tsp. olive oil

½ to ¾ cup minced onion

½ cup ea. diced carrots, green bell pepper, and corn (the last is optional but good)

1 tsp. minced garlic

1 tsp. cumin

1 can (2 oz.) chilies, chopped or 1 fresh jalapeño chopped

1 cup long-grain rice

2 to 2½ cups fat-free low-sodium chicken or vegetable broth

Salt to taste

1 can, approx. 15 oz. ea. drained rinsed canned beans of your choice: black, red, great northern, chickpeas, kidney, etc.

3 oz. fresh chopped greens

Heat olive oil in nonstick pan and sauté onion a few minutes. Add carrots, peppers, and corn. Stir. Add garlic, cumin, chilies, rice, 2 cups broth, and beans. Bring to a boil. Cover and lower to simmer for 15 minutes. Add greens and cook 5 minutes or until rice is cooked. Add more broth if necessary.

Calories: 389

Carbohydrates: 74 percent 72g

Fiber: 10g

Protein: 18 percent 18g

Fat: 8 percent 3.5g

Saturated Fat: 0.5g

This is another recipe that's great as it is. If necessary, up the energy levels with vegetable, fruit, and milk selections as above.

Asparagus and Pasta Stir Fry

Another great vegetarian option. Try other vegetables, such as snow peas, broccoli, carrots, Chinese cabbage, etc. Serve with fresh fruit salad, flat bread, skim or soy milk.

8 oz. whole-wheat or regular pasta, cooked

1 lb. asparagus

2 tsp. olive oil

1 tsp. garlic or more to taste

1 tsp. ginger or more to taste

1 large bunch green onions sliced, green and white parts

3–4 TB. low-sodium light soy sauce

$\frac{1}{8}$ tsp. red-pepper flakes or more to taste

1 tsp. sesame seed oil

Cut asparagus into small pieces. Heat olive oil and sauté asparagus until bright green, about two minutes. Add garlic, ginger, onions, soy, and red-pepper flakes. Stir and cook until fragrant, about two minutes. Stir in sesame oil. Pour over hot pasta and serve. Serves four.

Calories: 285

Carbohydrates: 66 percent 51g

Fiber: 10g

Protein: 19 percent 15g

Fat: 15 percent 5g

Saturated Fat: 1g

Sumptuous Smoothies

The following smoothie recipes are high in carbohydrates and low in protein and fat, which makes them great for drinking before events when time is short. They are also good sources of carbohydrates for postcompetition fueling. Except where noted, they can all be eaten less than one hour before an event or within 30 minutes after a practice or event.

These recipes are great as they are, but you can also use them as a departure point for your own recipes. Try any of the following suggestions for making your own smoothie sensations:

◆ Boost calcium in smoothies (power bars and snack mixes, too) with nonfat powdered milk. Start with a tablespoon or two and go from there.

◆ Use low-fat evaporated milk for a thick, rich-tasting smoothie.

- If you're lactose intolerant, try rice milk or soy in your smoothies.

- Soft silken tofu is a great addition to smoothies. It instantly makes them rich and creamy and is loaded with nutrients.

- Make your own fruit-on-the-bottom yogurt. Stir in 2 tablespoons fruit spread to 8 ounces vanilla yogurt.

- Mint isn't just for juleps! A few leaves of fresh mint give a blast of flavor and a refreshing taste to smoothies. Plus, it's a good digestive herb.

- Freeze it! Frozen fruit, peeled and cut up if necessary, is great for smoothies as it instantly thickens and chills them.

- Add a few gratings of fresh ginger to a smoothie for a sweet, pungent flavor that helps with nausea.

Most smoothies are plenty sweet on their own. If you have to sweeten them, choose natural sweeteners over sugar. Honey has twice the sweetening power of white sugar. Brown rice syrup and barley malt are other good natural sweeteners. Stevia, a natural herbal sweetener, is even sweeter—30 to several thousand times sweeter than sugar, depending on where it is grown. You can grow stevia or buy it in liquid or powder form.

Lite and Luscious Apricot Pineapple Smoothie

1 cup unsweetened pineapple juice

1 cup apricot nectar

1 cup fat-free vanilla ice cream or frozen yogurt

1 cup 2% milk

1 TB. honey

4 ice cubes

Blend until smooth. Serves four.

Calories: 160

Carbohydrates: 83 percent 34g

Fiber: 1g

Protein: 10 percent 4g

Fat: 7 percent 1.5g

Saturated Fat: 0.5g

Mango Mania

2 cups chopped mango

1 cup orange juice

$^1/_2$ cup soft silken tofu

2 TB. honey

4 ice cubes

Blend until smooth. Serves three.

Calories: 180

Carbohydrates: 89 percent 42g

Fiber: 2g

Protein: 5 percent 2g

Fat: 6 percent 1.5g

Saturated Fat: 0.0g

Protein Power Smoothie

You might need to reduce the fat slightly in this recipe by adding more ice cream per serving. The original recipe called for 1 cup of fat-free vanilla ice cream. You can make it with $1^1/_2$ cups or 2 cups, whichever you think is best.

$1^1/_2$ to 2 cups fat-free vanilla ice cream or frozen yogurt

1 cup 1% vanilla soy milk

2 TB. reduced-fat peanut butter

$^1/_2$ cup soft silken tofu

Blend until smooth. Serves two.

Calories: 330

Carbohydrates: 61 percent 53g

Fiber: 2g

Protein: 21 percent 18g

Fat: 18 percent 7g

Saturated Fat: 1g

Great for less than one hour before an event.

Great for postgame within 30 minutes after practice/event.

Triple Berry Smoothie

8 oz. low-fat fruit on the bottom yogurt, raspberry flavor

$^1/_3$ cup cranberry juice

1 cup raspberries

$^1/_2$ cup blueberries

4 ice cubes

Blend until smooth. Serves three.

Calories: 130

Carbohydrates: 80 percent 27g

Fiber: 3g

Protein: 12 percent 4g

Fat: 8 percent 1g

Saturated Fat: 0.5g

Wake-Up Call Smoothie

1 cup orange juice

1 cup strawberries, blackberries, or raspberries

1 cup chopped mango or papaya

1 banana, cut up

1 TB. honey or few drops stevia

4 ice cubes

Blend until smooth. Serves three.

Calories: 130

Carbohydrates: 94 percent 42g

Fiber: 3g

Protein: 3 percent 1g

Fat: 3 percent 0g less than 0.5g

Saturated Fat: 0g less than 0.5g

Three-Fruit Smoothie

1 ripe banana cut up

6 oz. frozen cranberry juice concentrate, thawed

1¼ cups orange juice

8 ice cubes

Blend until smooth. Serves three.

Calories: 200

Carbohydrates: 98 percent 50g

Fiber: 1g

Protein: 1 percent 0g

Fat: 1 percent 0g less than 0.5g

Saturated Fat: 0g less than 0.5g

Lemon Slushy Smoothie

2 cups lemon sherbet

1½ cups lemon-flavored sports drink

8 ice cubes

Blend everything. Serves four.

Calories: 125

Carbohydrates: 87 percent 28g

Fiber: 0g

Protein: 3 percent 1g

Fat: 10 percent 1.5g

Saturated Fat: 1g

Chocolate Lover's Frosty

1 cup skim milk

$^1/_4$ cup fat-free chocolate syrup

2 cups low-fat frozen chocolate yogurt

Blend everything until smooth. Serves three.

Calories: 246

Carbohydrates: 74 percent 48g

Fiber: 3g

Protein: 16 percent 11g

Fat: 9 percent 3g

Saturated Fat: 2g

Great for one to two hours before an event.

Great for postgame within 30 minutes after practice/event.

Double Chocolate Malted

1 cup skim milk

$^1/_4$ cup chocolate milk powder

2 cups fat-free chocolate ice cream or frozen yogurt

$^1/_2$ cup soft silken tofu

Blend everything. Makes three servings.

Calories: 260 calories

Carbohydrates: 78 percent 50g

Fiber: 2g

Protein: 17 percent 11g

Fat: 5 percent 1.5g

Saturated Fat: 0.5g

Great for one to two hours before an event.

Great for postgame within 30 minutes after practice/event.

Chocolate Malted Smoothie

1½ cups skim or 1% soy milk

2 cups fat-free vanilla or chocolate ice cream

¼ cup chocolate syrup

2 TB. malted milk powder

4 ice cubes

Blend everything. Serves three.

Calories: 293

Carbohydrates: 83 percent 61g

Fiber: 3g

Protein: 13 percent 10g

Fat: 4 percent 1.5g

Saturated Fat: 0.5g

Great for one to two hours before an event.

Great for postgame within 30 minutes after practice/event.

Strawberry Lemonade

3 cups lemonade

1 cup unsweetened frozen strawberries, thawed

4 ice cubes

Blend. Makes four servings.

Calories: 90

Carbohydrates: 98 percent 25g

Fiber: 1g

Protein: 2 percent 0g

Fat: 1 percent 0g

Saturated Fat: 0g

Great for less than one hour before practice/event.

Great after an event/practice within 30 minutes.

Quick-Fix Fruit Frappe

2 cups vanilla soy milk

1 ripe banana cut up

1 cup strawberries

1 tsp. vanilla

4 ice cubes

Sugar, honey, or sugar substitute to taste (start with 2 tsp.—optional)

Blend everything until smooth. Makes four servings.

Calories: 100

Carbohydrates: 81 percent 23g

Fiber: 2g

Protein: 9 percent 3g

Fat: 10 percent 1.5g

Saturated Fat: 0g

Formulated with 2 tsp. honey

Great for less than one hour before practice/event.

Great after an event/practice within 30 minutes.

Tropical Dream Smoothie

1 cup pineapple juice

1 banana cut up

$^1/_3$ cup nonfat instant dry powdered milk

1 tsp. vanilla

4 ice cubes

Sugar, honey, or sugar substitute to taste (optional—start with 3 TB.)

Blend. Makes two servings.

Calories: 260

Carbohydrates: 91 percent 63g

Fiber: 2g

Protein: 7 percent 5g

Fat: 2 percent 0g

Saturated Fat: 0g

Analyzed with 3 TB. honey

Great one to two hours before practice/event.

Great after an event/practice within 30 minutes.

Dawn Says

Ground flaxseed or flaxseed oil is a great addition to any smoothie. Flax is a rich source of omega-3 essential fatty acids, which helps our brains and may help to prevent irregular heartbeat, too. Flax also contains antioxidants and plant estrogens that may reduce cancer risk. And, it's an excellent source of fiber. Store seeds and oil in the refrigerator.

Berry Cherry Smoothie

1 cup 1% cherry or blueberry yogurt

$^1/_2$ cup cranberry juice

1 cup fresh or frozen blueberries

1 cup fresh pitted or frozen pitted cherries

4 ice cubes

Blend everything until smooth. Serves three.

Calories: 220

Carbohydrates: 81 percent 46g

Fiber: 3g

Protein: 11 percent 6g

Fat: 8 percent 2g

Saturated Fat: 1g

Great one to two hours before practice/event.

Great after an event/practice within 30 minutes.

Nutty Banana Smoothie

1 cup skim or 1% soy milk

1 TB. nonfat dry milk powder

2 TB. reduced-fat peanut butter

1 banana, cut up

2 tsp. honey

4 ice cubes

Blend until smooth. Serves two.

Calories: 210

Carbohydrates: 58 percent 32g

Fiber: 2g

Protein: 18 percent 10g

Fat: 24 percent 6g

Saturated Fat: 1g

Great two to three hours before practice/event.

Great after an event/practice within 30 minutes.

Peachy Keen Smoothie

8 oz. low-fat yogurt with fruit on the bottom, peach flavor

1 cup diced peaches

1 cup soy milk

2 TB. honey

4 ice cubes

1 TB. ground flaxseed

Blend until smooth. Serves three.

Calories: 191

Carbohydrates: 80 percent 39g

Fiber: 1.5g

Protein: 13 percent 7g

Fat: 7 percent 1.5g

Saturated Fat: 0.5g

Tangy Papaya Smoothie

1 cup diced papaya

1 banana, cut up

1 TB. flaxseed or wheat germ

1 cup orange-flavored sports drink

1 cup strawberries

4 ice cubes

Blend until smooth. Serves three.

Calories: 100

Carbohydrates: 84 percent 24g

Fiber: 4g

Protein: 5 percent 1.5g

Eat It Up!

Use a sugar substitute, soy, rice, or fat-free milk, fat-free and sugar-free ice creams and frozen yogurts, or fruits of your choice. Experiment and come up with your own "signature" recipe!

Fat: 6 percent 1.5g

Saturated Fat: 0.0g

Powering Up with Power Bars and Other Great Snacks

Go-the-Distance Trail Mix

Mix:

¹/₄ cup ea.:

Roasted pumpkin seeds

Roasted sunflower seeds

Soy nuts (your choice: plain, salted, or flavored)

Almonds

Dried Cranberries

Peanuts

Pistachios or Walnuts

Carob chips

Yogurt-covered raisins

Makes 2–14 cups. Serving size: ¹/₄ cup ea.; nine servings total

Calories: 197

Carbohydrates: 30 percent 15g

Fiber: 3g

Protein: 15 percent 7.5g

Fat: 56 percent 13g

Saturated Fat: 3g

This recipe by itself is too high in healthy fat for optimal performance. You can balance the fat by adding a 20-ounce sports drink and a fat-free yogurt to one serving of the mix.

You have a great snack two to three hours before practice or event.

For postgame you also have to have it mixed with high carbs for optimal recovery.

With a 20-ounce sports drink and yogurt

Calories: 494

Carbohydrates: 62 percent 77g

Fiber: 3g

Protein: 15 percent 18g

Fat: 23 percent 13g

Saturated Fat: 3g

World's Best Trail Mix 2

2¹/₂ cups round toasted oat cereal (like Cheerios)

¹/₂ cup soy nuts

¹/₂ cup chopped almonds or walnuts

¹/₂ cup unsweetened coconut

1¹/₂ cups dried fruit

¹/₂ cup raisins

¹/₂ cup sweetened condensed milk

Mix dry ingredients together. Pour milk over and stir to coat. Bake in preheated 275 degree oven on sprayed cookie sheet for 30–40 minutes, stirring every 15 minutes. Let cool. Makes about 6 cups mix. Serves 12. Serving size: ¹/₂ cup each.

Calories: 243

Carbohydrates: 58 percent 38g

Fiber: 6g

Protein: 12 percent 8g

Fat: 30 percent 9g

Saturated Fat: 4g

Good three to four hours before an event/practice. If you add a 20-ounce sports drink to a serving of this Trail Mix you can bump it up to two to three hours before a practice or event. Postgame you can have with or without a sports drink.

With a 20-ounce sports drink

Calories: 393

Carbohydrates: 73 percent 75g

Fiber: 6g

Protein: 8 percent 8g

Fat: 19 percent 9g

Saturated Fat: 4g

Caramel Cranberry Crunch

4 cups popped corn

1 TB. flaxseed

1/4 cup caramel ice cream topping, heated in microwave

1 cup Craisins

Mix popcorn and flax. Pour topping over, stirring to coat. Bake in preheated 250 degree oven for 30–40 minutes. Cool. Makes 4 cups. Serves four. Serving size: 1 cup each.

Caramel Cranberry Popcorn Balls

Follow above recipe but don't bake. Pack mixture into sprayed 1 cup measure, remove, and form into balls. Makes 4 balls. Serving size: 1 ball. These balls stay chewy if wrapped.

Calories: 219

Carbohydrates: 81 percent 45g

Fiber: 3g

Protein: 4 percent 2g

Fat: 4 percent 4g

Saturated Fat: 0g

Great one to two hours before practice/event.

Great after an event/practice within 30 minutes.

Yummy Maple Granola

$1/3$ cup maple syrup

$1/4$ cup Canola oil

1 tsp. vanilla

2 cups old-fashioned oatmeal

1 cup dried diced fruit

Mix syrup, oil, and vanilla. Pour over oatmeal and mix well. Spread on cookie sheet and bake in preheated 350 degree oven for 10 minutes. Let cool and mix with dried fruit. Makes 3 cups. Serves six. Serving size: $1/2$ cup each.

Calories: 280

Carbohydrates: 59 percent 42g

Fiber: 4g

Protein: 7 percent 5g

Fat: 35 percent 11g

Saturated Fat: 1g

This recipe by itself is a little too high in fat for optimal performance levels. You can add a 20-ounce sports drink to the mix for a well-balanced snack two to three hours before your event or practice. This is also a good recipe if you don't like to eat much the day of competition. You should also have a sports drink or a fruit juice (100 percent juice, of course) with it for post game recovery within 30 minutes of activity.

With a 20-ounce sports drink

Calories: 430

Carbohydrates: 73 percent 80g

Fiber: 4g

Protein: 4 percent 5g

Fat: 23 percent 11g

Saturated Fat: 1g

Honey Apricot Power Bars

2¼ cups quick-cooking oatmeal

½ cup chopped soy nuts

¼ cup chopped nuts

⅓ cup light tub margarine, 4.5g fat per tsp.

½ cup packed brown sugar

¼ cup honey, malt, or rice syrup

1½ tsp. cinnamon

1½ cups chopped apricots or other dried fruit

½ cup dry nonfat milk powder

1 TB. wheat germ

1 cup corn cereal squares, crushed

Preheat oven to 350 degrees. Pour oatmeal, soy nuts, and nuts onto cookie sheet. Bake 10 minutes. Set aside. Combine margarine, brown sugar, honey, and cinnamon in large pan. Cook over medium heat until mixture boils. Pour toasted oat mixture, apricots, milk powder, wheat germ, and corn cereal into honey mixture. Blend. Pour into foil-lined and sprayed 8"×8" pan. Press mixture into pan. Bake 12–15 minutes. Remove from oven and after mixture cools remove foil and cut into 24 bars. Serving size: 1 bar.

Calories: 220

Carbohydrates: 67 percent 38g

Fiber: 2g

Protein: 9 percent 5g

Fat: 24 percent 6g

Saturated Fat: 1g

Great two to three hours before practice/event. Also good after an event/practice within 30 minutes; better if you gulp it down with at least 10 ounces of a sports drink, V8 Splash, or one banana.

Marshmallow Granola Energizers

3 TB. margarine

3 cups mini marshmallows, about 6–7 oz.

1 tsp. vanilla

1 tsp. ground cinnamon

Mix:

2 cups low-fat granola

1 cup rice chex cereal, crushed

1 cup salted or unsalted soy nuts, crushed

$^1/_4$ cup diced dried fruit (optional but good)

Melt margarine and marshmallows. Add vanilla and cinnamon and stir. Pour granola, rice chex, and soy nuts into mixture. Blend well. Press into foil-lined and sprayed 8"×8" pan. Cool and cut into 8 squares. Serving size: 1 square.

Calories: 230

Carbohydrates: 67 percent 41g

Fiber: 2g

Protein: 8 percent 5g

Fat: 25 percent 7g

Saturated Fat: 1.5g

Great two to three hours before practice/event. Good after an event or practice within 30 minutes; better if you drink it down with skim milk, 100 percent fruit juice, or a sports drink.

Endurance Bars

$^1/_2$ cup brown rice syrup

$^1/_4$ cup honey

$^1/_3$ cup low-fat peanut butter

Mix:

2 cups crispy rice cereal

1 cup grape nuts cereal

$^1/_4$ cup wheat germ

$^1/_4$ cup soy nuts, crushed**

$^1/_4$ cup dried mixed fruit, chopped if necessary

1 TB. flax meal (optional)

Bring rice syrup, honey, and peanut butter to a boil over medium heat on stove or microwave on high two minutes or just until mixture boils. Pour over cereal mixture. Stir until well blended. Press into foil-lined and sprayed 8"×8" pan. Cool. Cut into 16 bars. Serving size: 1 bar.

**To crush any nuts or cereal easily, place in zip-lock bag and hit with mallet or bottom of saucepan.

Calories: 159

Carbohydrates: 70 percent 29g

Fiber: 2g

Protein: 13 percent 5g

Fat: 17 percent 3g

Saturated Fat: 0.6g

Great one to two hours before practice or event.

Great after practice/event within 30 minutes.

The Least You Need to Know

- ◆ What you eat before competition must provide you with adequate carbohydrate energy, especially if you compete in the morning following an overnight fast.

- ◆ Decreasing protein and fat levels in foods a day prior to an event will help fuel optimal performance.

- ◆ Flaxseed oil, which is a rich source of omega-3 essential fatty acids, is a great addition to smoothies.

- ◆ Adding a sports drink or yogurt can help boost the carbohydrate levels of recipes that are higher in protein and fat.

Part 4

Athletes In All Shapes and Sizes

Everyone's body works in basically the same way. Yet, depending on gender, age, and a few other factors, nutritional needs can vary widely. Men rarely need iron supplementation; women often do. Kids need more calories than adults, and they need to eat more fat, too. Vegetarians have nutritional concerns that are different from those of people who eat meat. Because they generally eat less than younger people do, seniors often lack important nutrients like calcium and B vitamins that could both boost their strength and stamina and protect them from age-related diseases and disorders.

If you're a parent concerned about teaching your kids the benefits of good nutrition, a senior wanting the inside scoop on how to eat to increase your energy, a vegetarian looking for ways to increase iron consumption, or you're simply looking for nutritional guidance tailored to the specific needs of male and female athletes, you've come to the right place.

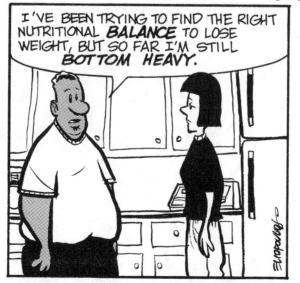

Chapter 17

Nutrition for the Female Athlete

In This Chapter

- ◆ Starving for excellence
- ◆ Understanding the "female athlete triad"
- ◆ Turning bad eating habits into good ones
- ◆ Supplements to support healthy bones

Women were born to be active, and since the dawn of history they have been. When the men were out hunting, women shouldered the main responsibilities for providing the other foods for their tribes. In fact, women were the original beasts of burden when it came to ensuring the survival of their families. All that stuff about the "weaker sex" came along much later. And, fortunately, it's pretty much been wiped out today.

There have been some great female athletes throughout the centuries, but there's nothing to match the current numbers of women who participate in sports. Thanks to the passage of Title IX in 1972, women were given the chance to participate in sports with roughly the same levels of support as men receive.

Today, women are going for the gold more and more, in gyms and workout facilities as well as arenas and playing fields. And they're learning that food can be their friend, rather than their foe, when it comes to fueling their performances.

The Unique Needs of the Female Athlete

Sports nutrition has important benefits for all active people, but it plays an even more important role when it comes to active women. Women, of course, have different builds than men. However, they have physiological differences that go beyond this. As a rule, they carry more fat and less muscle than men do. This extra fat both protects the sex organs and plays a role in nurturing the fetus during pregnancy. Being equipped for childbearing plays a huge rule in how a woman's body functions throughout her life and in her nutritional needs. When a woman is active, it's vital that her nutrition is adequate in both arenas.

Just like men, active women usually need to increase their energy intake to fuel optimal performance. However, they often resist doing so because of concerns over their appearance and their size—concerns that are often a result of the sports they compete in.

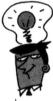

Eat It Up!

To put it mildly, women's sports have "come a long way, baby." In 1998, 2.1 million young women were participating in high school sports programs, a huge rise from the approximately 300,000 females who competed in 1971, the year before the passage of Title IX.

In general, women tend to excel at sports that are high on the aesthetic scale—activities like gymnastics, ballet, and other forms of dance, figure skating, diving, rowing, and running. These sports put a high premium on appearance. Some are actually referred to as "weight-dependent" sports, as what a woman weighs can make a huge difference in her performance. To be competitive, women who compete in these sports often restrict their calories to the point where they don't eat enough to keep them healthy, much less fuel good performance.

The demands of competing at the top levels in these sports put female athletes at risk for developing eating disorders including anorexia nervosa, anorexia athletica (exercising to excess to keep body weight down), and bulimia nervosa. However, it's not just elite athletes who are at risk for these disorders. Sadly, the number of women—active and not—of all ages who suffer from them is steadily increasing. At a time when we know so much about nutrition's role in preventing disease and maintaining good health, more women than ever before are putting their health in danger by eating inadequate diets. What's more, these problems aren't related to women who are starving themselves to stay thin. Normal-sized and overweight women suffer from nutritional deficiencies as well, often caused by confusion over conflicting advice as to what they should be eating. The diet of the week often turns into the eating disorder of the year.

Missing Minerals

What all women are at risk for is lower-than-optimal levels of two important micro-nutrients: calcium and iron. All women need at least 1,000 mg of calcium and 15 mg of iron daily just to meet their minimum requirements of these important minerals; however, many women don't come close to these levels. The lack of calcium, of course, can lead to osteoporosis, which we'll discuss in more detail later in this chapter.

Iron is the other important nutrient that many women are deficient in. According to the National Institutes of Health, approximately 20 percent of all women are believed to be *iron deficient* or *anemic*. These rates are higher in adolescent females, pregnant women, and female athletes. Studies show that between one third to one half of athletic women have low iron stores.

Foodie _____

Iron deficiency or ane-mia is defined as a condition that occurs when the body's iron stores are too low to allow normal functioning.

Not having enough iron in the body is a real problem when it comes to athletic performance. When iron levels are low, the blood's ability to carry oxygen to the cells falls along with it. As oxygen levels diminish, the muscles literally begin to suffocate. In technical terms, they lose their aerobic capacity. In other words, they can't function like they should.

As previously discussed, iron comes in two forms: plant based and animal based. Because many female athletes don't eat enough calories to start with, they don't get enough dietary iron from either source. But there's an even greater problem when it comes to iron, because the body doesn't absorb both forms equally.

The most easily absorbed form of iron is heme iron, which is found in animal protein and particularly in red meat. Nonheme iron comes with some baggage—fiber—that makes it harder to absorb. Because of this, you have to eat more foods that contain nonheme iron to get the same amount that you would if you ate meat. Or you can boost your absorption of nonheme iron by eating a little meat along with those veggies and grains. The problem is, many female athletes also aren't meat eaters. Even if they are, they often don't eat enough of it to supply the amount of iron they need.

When iron levels get low, both health and athletic performance can be compromised. Athletes who are low in iron can suffer from the following problems:

- Shortness of breath

- Headache

Eat It Up!

Women who participate in endurance sports such as distance running, or who are vegetarians, are at even greater risk for developing iron deficiency. If you're in either group, you need to be particularly careful about what you eat to make sure you get enough iron.

- Decreased appetite

- Loss of endurance

- Chronic fatigue

The cure, of course, is to increase the consumption of foods that contain iron, and, if necessary, to take supplemental iron. Unfortunately, most women who are iron deficient aren't aware of the problem, so they don't do anything about it. They continue to eat a diet that lacks important nutrients. As they do, they set themselves up for some truly serious problems.

Foodie

Amenorrhea is the absence of menstruation that lasts for longer than six months, or a decrease in the frequency of menstrual periods.

The Female Athlete Triad

Eating an inadequate diet—one that lacks important nutrients and calories—is an early indicator of what is called the "female athlete triad"—a syndrome of disordered eating, *amenorrhea*, and osteoporosis that is occurring with increased frequency among physically active girls and women.

Recognizing the Syndrome

The female athlete triad typically begins when female control body weight by adopting one or more of the following behaviors:

- Eating erratically—skipping meals and/or avoiding certain foods

- Reducing food intake

- Making poor food choices

- Using appetite suppressants and diet pills

- Using laxatives, diuretics, or enemas

- Vomiting after meals

High-intensity exercise beyond what is called for by their particular sport or activity may also play a role.

As previously mentioned, the decrease in calories often leads to nutritional deficiencies and especially deficiencies in calcium and iron. Performance levels often decline because these women simply don't get enough energy and nutrients. Their health declines as well, with gastrointestinal problems and hypothermia, or lower-than-normal body temperatures, being common.

As this pattern of poor eating and excessive exercise continues, estrogen levels decline, causing menstrual periods to either become less frequent or stop completely. Lower estrogen levels can also reduce calcium levels in the bones, as the body needs normal levels of this hormone for optimal calcium absorption. As calcium levels drop, bones lose thickness and strength, resulting in low bone mass and osteoporosis.

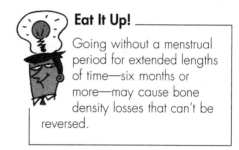

Eat It Up!

Going without a menstrual period for extended lengths of time—six months or more—may cause bone density losses that can't be reversed.

Although these habits are a concern for all women, they're a particular problem for young female athletes. Lower-than-normal estrogen and calcium levels disrupt the growing process of the bones, which means that they might never develop as they should. Bringing estrogen and calcium levels back up can halt bone loss and eventually rebuild it, although some experts believe that bone strength and density will always be somewhat less than what they should be in these women.

Women who are most likely to be at risk for developing the female athlete triad syndrome include these groups:

◆ High school and intercollegiate athletes who are highly competitive in endurance sports, such as distance running, race-walking, bicycling, rowing, etc.

◆ Girls and women who participate in activities that emphasize appearance and leanness, such as gymnastics, ballet, figure skating, diving, rowing, horseback riding, cycling, and track and field; or sports like rowing which involve weight classfications.

◆ Noncompetitive but still physically active girls and women who diet and exercise to excess.

If allowed to continue, the behaviors that create the female athletic triad can have serious consequences. Not being able to compete at optimal levels are the least of the problems that these women face. They also run the risk of having difficulties bearing children and of suffering crippling bone fractures.

While awareness of the female athlete triad has substantially increased since the syndrome was identified, it remains a problem as the symptoms can be difficult to detect. Most of the girls—and women—who are at the highest risk for developing these problems look perfectly healthy—in fact, they're often the envy of their friends because they look so fit and lean. An x-ray of their spine, however, would tell another story. The spinal bone density of a young athlete who has stopped or never started having menstrual periods can resemble that of a 70-year-old woman.

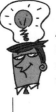

Eat It Up!

According to researchers, the incidence of eating disorders in female athletes ranges from 16 to 72 percent, compared to 5 to 10 percent in the general population. Menstrual irregularities are also more prevalent among women who participate in varsity athletics, with 28 percent of them experiencing no or few periods.

Preventing the Syndrome

Unfortunately, as long as there are sports that place a high premium on appearance and weight, there will be women running the risk of damaging their health when they compete in them. For the women who do enjoy these activities and want to do them, it's essential to develop good nutritional habits early on to avoid long-term health problems. The food they eat needs to be as nutrient-packed as possible. If eating continues to be a problem, it's a good idea to consult with a sports nutritionist who can assess current food habits and needs and develop an eating program based on them.

Basic Nutrition for Active Women

Many female athletes don't take in enough calories to support their nutritional needs, even when they play sports that enable them to maintain a healthy weight.

Dawn Says

Sedentary women can generally eat around 1,600 calories a day to maintain their weight. Active women—those women who work out on a regular basis and in general lead an active lifestyle—usually need at least another 600 calories to keep them feeling right. Extremely active women and competitive athletes can eat as much as 3,000 calories a day or more, depending on their size and activity level.

Some women who lead active lifestyles may eat enough calories, but they don't eat foods that provide optimum nutrition. Because of this, all active women should take nutritional supplementation in the form of a good multivitamin/multimineral. It doesn't make up for eating right, but it does add a layer of insurance against nutritional deficiencies.

The following guidelines will also help bring nutrient levels up and improve performance:

- Eat 45 to 70 percent of calories from complex carbohydrates—vegetables, grains, fruit, etc.

- High-quality protein should comprise 10 to 30 percent of calories. If you're building muscle, you'll need to eat at the higher end of this range. Women in their 30s and beyond should consider getting some of their protein in the form of soy products, as they can also help cushion the hormonal changes associated with perimenopause.

- Calcium intake should be between 800 and 1,200 mg daily. If you're experiencing menstrual irregularities, boost your intake to 1,500 mg daily. If you don't consume dairy products, take supplements to reach these levels. Drink orange juice when eating foods that contain calcium to boost the absorption of this important mineral.

- Iron intake should be 15 mg a day. The best sources are animal protein; adding a little meat to vegetable dishes will also aid the absorption of nonheme iron contained in these foods. If iron deficiency is a concern, supplementation may be necessary. Vitamin C also boosts iron absorption.

- Drink 8 to 10 glasses of water a day. For hydration guidelines for competing or working out, turn to Chapter 3.

- Minimize your intake of foods that are high in fat, sodium, and sugar. If you're not eating that many calories to begin with, these foods can quickly push you beyond your intake levels. However, it is important to get adequate levels of healthy fats, and the eating plan outlined here does allow for this. For a refresher on what they are, turn to Chapter 9.

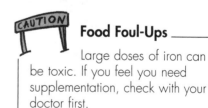

Food Foul-Ups

Large doses of iron can be toxic. If you feel you need supplementation, check with your doctor first.

Sample Menus for Active Women

Dawn designed the following menus to provide optimal nutrient balances for five different calorie levels. Each menu contains about 55 to 60 percent carbohydrates, 18 to 20 percent protein, and 20 to 25 percent fat. They do not reflect pre- and postgame meals and snacks. Eighteen hundred calories is the minimum amount that active/athletic teenagers and women should eat. If less is necessary, consult with a dietitian who emphasizes sports nutrition. Consider these menus as a guide. Most athletes eat at least four times a day. Some eat six times a day. The best approach is to tailor your program to your specific schedule and exercise plan.

1,800 Calorie Menu

Breakfast 7:30 A.M. to 9:30 A.M.

16 oz. skim milk

2 whole eggs

Egg whites

$^{1}/_{2}$ cup oatmeal; you can add flax mill or oil if you only use egg whites

1 cup blueberries

16 oz. water

Vitamin and mineral supplements

Lunch 11:30 A.M. to 1:30 P.M.

2 slices low-cal, high-fiber bread or

1 slice Brownberry bread

3 oz. turkey–lean

2 cups snow peas

16 oz. water

Afternoon Snack 2:30 P.M. to 4:30 P.M.

$1^{1}/_{2}$ cups low-fat cottage cheese

1 cup canned or 2 whole peaches

16 oz. water

Evening Meal 5:30 P.M. to 7:30 P.M.

6 oz. grilled teriyaki chicken

1½ cups cooked broccoli; use a nontrans-fatty acid margarine sparingly

16 oz. water

Vitamin and mineral supplements

2,100 Calorie Menu

Breakfast 7:30 A.M. to 9:30 A.M.

16 oz. skim milk

2 whole eggs

4 egg whites

1 cup oatmeal; can add flax oil or mill if you use only egg whites

2 cups blueberries

16 oz. water

Vitamin and mineral supplement

Lunch 11:30 A.M. to 1:30 P.M.

2 slices Brownberry Bread

5 oz. turkey–lean

2 cups snow peas

1 apple

16 oz. water

Afternoon Snack 2:30 P.M. to 4:30 P.M.

2½ cups low-fat cottage cheese

½ cup canned or 1 whole peaches

16 oz. water

Evening Meal 5:30 P.M. to 7:30 P.M.

6 oz. grilled teriyaki chicken

1¹/₂ cups cooked broccoli; use a nontrans-fatty acid margarine sparingly

3 cups mixed greens

2 TB. low-fat dressing

16 oz. water

Vitamin and mineral supplement

2,400 Calorie Menu

Breakfast 7:30 A.M. to 9:30 A.M.

16 oz. skim milk

3 egg whites

1 whole egg white

1¹/₂ cups oatmeal with flax oil or meal

2 cups blueberries

20 oz. water

Vitamin and mineral supplements

Lunch 11:30 A.M. to 1:30 P.M.

4 slices Brownberry Bread

5 oz. turkey–lean

2 cups snow peas

1 apple

20 oz. water

Afternoon Snack 2:30 P.M. to 4:30 P.M.

2 cups low-fat cottage cheese

16 oz. skim milk

$^{1}/_{2}$ cup canned or 1 whole peaches

20 oz. water

Evening Meal 5:30 P.M. to 7:30 P.M.

6 oz. grilled teriyaki chicken

$1^{1}/_{2}$ cups cooked broccoli; use a nontrans-fatty acid margarine sparingly

3 cups mixed greens

2 TB. fat-free or low-fat dressing

20 oz. water

Vitamin and mineral supplements

2,700 Calorie Menu

Breakfast 7:30 A.M. to 9:30 A.M.

20 oz. skim milk

3 egg whites

1 whole egg

2 cups oatmeal

2 cup blueberries

20 oz. water

Vitamin and mineral supplements

Lunch 11:30 A.M. to 1:30 P.M.

4 slices Brownberry bread

6 oz. turkey–lean

1 sliced tomato

2 cups snow peas

3 apples

20 oz. water

Afternoon Snack 2:30 P.M. to 4:30 P.M.

2 cups low-fat cottage cheese

16 oz. skim milk

1 cup canned or 2 whole peaches

20 oz. water

Evening Meal 5:30 P.M. to 7:30 P.M.

6 oz. grilled teriyaki chicken

1½ cups cooked broccoli; use a nontrans-fatty acid margarine sparingly

3 cups mixed greens

2 TB. fat-free or low-fat dressing

20 oz. water

Vitamin and mineral supplements

3,000 Calorie Menu

Breakfast 7:30 A.M. to 9:30 A.M.

24 oz. skim milk

3 egg whites

1 whole egg

2½ cups oatmeal

2 cups blueberries

20 oz. water

Vitamin and mineral supplements

Lunch 11:30 A.M. to 1:30 P.M.

6 oz. tuna fish mixed with brown rice with hot sauce or salsa

2½ cups brown rice

3½ cups grapes

2 cups radishes

1 cup celery

16 oz. water

Afternoon Snack 2:30 P.M. to 4:30 P.M.

2 cups low-fat cottage cheese

16 oz. skim milk

1 cup canned or 2 whole peaches

20 oz. water

Evening Meal 5:30 P.M. to 7:30 P.M.

7 oz. grilled teriyaki chicken

2 cups cooked broccoli; use a nontrans-fatty acid margarine sparingly

3 cups mixed greens

2 TB. fat-free or low-fat dressing

20 oz. water

Vitamin and mineral supplements

Nutrition for the Pregnant Athlete

Pregnancy used to mean hanging up your athletic shoes for nine months, plus some time afterward to take care of your new little one. Times have definitely changed and they've definitely changed for the better. Not only do many women continue to stay active and even compete for at least part of their pregnancies, the general wisdom today is that it's good to do so as long as mother and child are in good health. Keeping active while pregnant, and following a good nutritional program, can go a long way to ensure lifelong good health for baby and mom.

When you're pregnant, you're the food supply for your baby. If you don't eat right, your baby won't get the nutrients it needs to thrive.

According to the March of Dimes, pregnant women should increase their daily food portions to include the following:

- Six to eleven servings of breads and other whole grains
- Three to five servings of vegetables

- Two to four servings of fruits

- Four to six servings of milk and milk products

- Three to four servings of meat and protein foods

If you're maintaining anything close to your usual activity level, you'll want to eat on the high side of these recommendations.

In addition, be sure to drink at least six to eight glasses of water a day. You should be doing this anyway, but drinking lots of fluids while you're pregnant is even more important. Studies have shown that dehydration increases the risk of premature contractions and early delivery. So keep those fluids coming! Aim for a minimum of eight large glasses of water a day. Keep a full water bottle with you at all times.

CAUTION **Food Foul-Ups** _____

It used to be believed that when a woman didn't eat well during pregnancy, her fetus would draw on her reserves to meet its needs. Although this is true when it comes to calcium, as the body will take this nutrient from its bones to sustain the needs of the developing baby, research has shown that babies born to mothers who didn't follow good nutritional practices are more likely to be premature, small, and unhealthy.

Some pregnant women find it difficult to stay active due to low carbohydrate intake. Not only does your body burn carbohydrates faster when you're pregnant, exercise also burns carbs. Combine the two and you run the risk of having low blood sugar when you work out and of developing harmful ketones which can cause fetal ketosis. Taking in enough carbs will prevent this problem.

As previously mentioned, anemia is another problem for many pregnant women. Since it hampers the blood's ability to carry oxygen, it also can have a big impact on your ability to exercise and how you feel when you do. To avoid it, be sure to eat an iron-rich diet, take extra vitamin C with meals to increase iron absorption, and take iron supplements if your doctor prescribes them.

The Least You Need to Know

- Active women usually need to increase their energy intake to fuel optimal performance. However, they often resist doing so because of concerns over their appearance and their size.

♦ Since female athletes often restrict calorie levels, the food they eat needs to supply optimal nutrition.

♦ Sedentary women can generally eat around 1,600 calories a day to maintain their weight. Active women usually need at least another 600 calories to keep feeling right.

♦ Almost all women can benefit from paying close attention to their calcium and iron intake. Supplementation of both vital nutrients may be necessary if dietary intake is low.

Nutrition for the Male Athlete

In This Chapter

- ◆ The inside story on men's eating habits
- ◆ How to make healthy convenience-food choices
- ◆ Best pantry choices for cooking-challenged men
- ◆ A sample eating plan for athletes and active men

Men, relatively speaking, have it pretty easy when it comes to nutrition. As a rule, the differences between the sexes enable men to eat more than women can. Because they can eat more, they don't run as great a risk of incurring nutrient-related health problems like women do.

Nutrition for active men and male athletes pretty much boils down to the basics: eating nutrient-dense foods, watching fat and protein intake, and staying hydrated. That sounds pretty easy, right? Unfortunately, lots of guys find it hard to do.

The Shape of Things for Guys

Not to pound too hard on the men here, but many of them are pretty clueless when it comes to nutrition basics. On the plus side, they also tend to have fewer issues with food than women do. Emotional eating isn't much of a problem for men. Neither do they use food as a reward as much as women do. Some men, however, can get pretty hung up on body image, or they compete in sports that are weight dependent like wrestling, body building, running, and gymnastics. When they do, eating problems can and do erupt.

Although eating disorders like anorexia or bulimia are more often associated with women, men suffer from them, too. Competitive wrestlers often have to diet stringently to make weight. Gymnasts, bodybuilders, and runners put a high premium on low body fat levels as well. It's easy for these guys to get into an ongoing cycle of bingeing and purging between events.

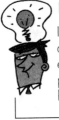

Eat It Up!

It's estimated that 1 to 5 percent of all men have unhealthy eating behaviors that are serious enough to qualify as eating disorders. Of the people diagnosed with eating disorders, 10 to 15 percent are men. The majority of them—more than 75 percent—binge eat, meaning that they gorge impulsively or continuously. The rest have bulimia or anorexia.

Many men view eating as something that they have to do, not as something they necessarily want to do. The actual act of eating doesn't give them that much pleasure. For this reason, men tend to eat on the run more than women do. Instead of giving themselves a constant source of energy by fueling their bodies throughout the day, they're also more likely to eat when they realize they're hungry.

Preparing meals, which is something that many women enjoy, is a nightmare for lots of guys. Unless they're taught how to do it at a young age, they try to avoid it at all costs because they simply don't know how to cook. If they're living by themselves, they eat prepackaged food when they're at home—your basic "man and a can" program. Or they rely on easy-to-prepare foods like protein shakes and skillet meals that they can whip up in a hurry. Spending hours slaving over a special dish? Waiting a half-hour for something to simmer or bake? Not in the game plan for most men.

While the nutritional needs of men and women aren't that different, how they eat is. When putting together an eating plan for men, it's important to find ways to make it easy for them to choose healthy food regardless of how they take it in. Eating out of a can isn't necessarily the end of the world. It all depends on what's in that can.

Eating Right, Guy Style

Whether you like to cook or not, the basics remain the basics when it comes to what you eat. You have to:

◆ Eat enough to keep you going.

◆ Choose your nutrients from a variety of food groups.

◆ Keep fat and sweets intake low (as a rule, though, you can eat more fat than women can).

◆ Watch your protein intake. Most men eat far too much. Even if you're trying to put on muscle, chances are pretty good that you don't need to eat much more protein, if any, than you're already taking in.

◆ Drink fluids to keep hydration levels where they should be. Eight 8-ounce glasses of the wet stuff a day is the minimum. You'll need more if you drink caffeinated beverages or alcohol, which dehydrate the body.

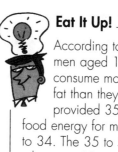

Eat It Up!

According to researchers, men aged 19 to 50 years consume more calories and fat than they should. Fat provided 35 percent of food energy for men aged 19 to 34. The 35 to 50 set ate a whopping 38 percent of their total daily calories in fat.

Men need to pay particular attention to their levels of fat intake because of its relationship to heart disease and cancer. High fat intake is a known contributor to both. If men depend on meat and dairy to meet their protein needs, their diets are almost guaranteed to be too high in fat. Switching to plant-based sources of protein will drop fat intake and boost the intake of dietary fiber, which many experts believe can protect against heart disease, colon cancer, hypertension, and gallstones. It will also increase levels of important antioxidants like beta carotene, vitamin C, and vitamin E.

When it comes to eating right, the way men eat can actually work to their advantage. Since they don't like to prepare food, they're more likely to reach for whole foods—raw fruit and raw vegetables—if they're handy. Lots of guys like to chow down on a bowl of cereal and milk when hunger hits. Make that cereal a whole-grain product, substitute skim or low-fat milk for higher-fat versions, and throw a sliced banana or some berries on it, and you've got the basis for a good meal.

It's also possible to eat healthily when you depend on convenience foods when you're eating at home. Protein bars and shakes aren't be-all, end-all when it comes to getting all the nutrients you need, but there is nothing wrong with including them in a meal plan if you like them. There are even protein drinks ready-made in a can that you can use if you don't feel like powering up your blender.

When it comes to other convenience foods—canned food, frozen food, and the like—knowing how to read Nutrition Facts labels can make the difference between an eating program that contains optimal nutrients and one that's too high in the things you don't need—sodium, sugars, protein, and fat. There are plenty of healthy convenience foods out there. You just need to learn how to find them. For a refresher on how to read food labels, turn to Chapter 4.

Stocking the Guy's Pantry

Making it easy to make good food choices means having healthy food on hand. Whether you're single, living with someone, or married, it's to your benefit to have a stash of healthy food around to grab when you need to eat. Here's a list to choose from:

♦ Tuna or other canned fish, such as sardines or mackerel

♦ Peanut butter

♦ Whole-wheat bread (keep it in the refrigerator or freezer and it won't get moldy)

♦ Canned beans. Rinse them before using to lower sodium levels. Nonfat refried beans are also a good choice.

♦ Canned soup or soup in a cup. Choose low-fat, low-sodium products.

♦ Whole-wheat crackers. Again, choose low-fat, low-sodium products whenever possible.

♦ Milk. Choose low-fat or skim.

♦ Lean meat. Buy packets of presliced meat for sandwiches.

♦ Protein powder and bars. Choose products that are low in fat.

♦ Eggs. They're an excellent source of protein, and a convenient one, especially if you cook up enough hard-boiled eggs to keep you going for a few days. If you're concerned about cholesterol, dump the yolks and just eat the whites, or eat just half the yolk. Egg substitutes are a good alternative.

♦ Fresh or frozen vegetables. Choose a variety of different types for optimal nutrition.

♦ Fresh or frozen fruit. Choose whole fruit over fruit juice for a fiber boost.

♦ Nonfat cottage cheese. It's one of the best protein foods out there. If you don't like the taste of nonfat cottage cheese, buy low-fat and nonfat cottage cheese and mix them together.

♦ Yogurt. Watch the sugar content here, as many yogurt products are high in it.

♦ Potatoes. They're a great source of carbohydrates and are easy to prepare if you have a microwave.

♦ Whole-grain products such as oatmeal, brown rice, whole-wheat pasta, cereal, etc.

Later in this chapter, you'll find excerpts from an eating program that was developed for a professional baseball player and that uses all of these foods.

> **Dawn Says**
>
> Three of the best investments a guy can make for his nutritional health are an indoor grill (think George Foreman), a microwave, and a blender. You can do just about anything with these appliances. When you're pushed for time, slap a chicken breast on that grill, defrost some vegetables, and add a grain-based carbohydrate of some type—maybe some leftover pasta or bread. Voilà! Instant dinner.

Supplements for Men

Although men usually eat more than women, they generally still fall short on vitamins and minerals because they don't often eat the right types of food. For example, researchers have found that middle-aged men are often low in vitamin B6 and vitamin E because they don't eat enough whole grains and vegetables. It's always advisable to ensure that you do get enough of the nutrients you need through a high-quality multivitamin/mineral supplement.

Supplementation plus eating a diet that is rich in whole grains, vegetables, and fruit can also boost consumption of some other nutrients that are important to male health, including these:

♦ Lycopene. There's evidence that this powerful phytochemical antioxidant may help prevent prostate cancer, heart disease, and other serious diseases, including other forms of cancer. It's found in red tomatoes, processed tomato products, and watermelon.

♦ Selenium. This micronutrient may also reduce the incidence of prostate cancer. Good sources include brazil nuts, fish, shellfish, chicken, wheat germ, brown rice, oatmeal, and eggs.

◆ Antioxidants such as vitamin C, vitamin E, and various bioflavonoids, shown to be important for cardiovascular health.

◆ Calcium. Although osteoporosis isn't as much of a problem for men as it is for women, it is still a concern, especially as men grow older and their ability to absorb it decreases.

Putting It All Together

The following nutrition program is excerpted from one that Dawn put together for one of her celebrity clients—a professional baseball player who wanted to lose body fat and gain muscle. It's a good example of an easy-to-follow eating program that requires minimal meal preparation yet delivers optimal nutrition.

Goals: Gain 10 pounds of muscle

Exercise with a personal trainer 5–6 times per week

Follow a sports nutrition daily plan

Only gain 2 pounds of weight a week

Measure body fat every 4–6 weeks

Weigh yourself weekly

No skipping meals

Nutrient servings required daily

Carbohydrates/Grains	22 servings
Fruit	8 servings
Vegetables	6 servings
Milk/Dairy	6 servings
Meat/Protein	18 servings

For approximately 4,000 calories a day, mainly from carbohydrates in the morning and lunch time.

To make this 3,500 calories a day:

Carbohydrates/Grains	19 servings
Fruit	7 servings

Vegetables	6 servings
Milk/Dairy	5 servings
Meat/Protein	16 servings

To make this 3,000 calories a day:

Carbohydrates/grains	16 servings
Fruits	6 servings
Vegetables	6 servings
Milk/Dairy	4 servings
Meat/Protein	14 servings

These calories still need to be adjusted depending on the scale and body fat measurements.

Based on this athlete's profile, he needed to eat 5,400 calories a day, but putting him on a plan that called for this much food right away could have caused him to gain body fat in the first three weeks. For this reason, he was started at 3,500 calories a day, which would be readjusted in about four to six weeks after body fat and muscle mass results were measured.

This athlete was currently eating a diet that contained 57 percent carbohydrates, 23 percent protein, and 20 percent fat. These values would change as his caloric value increased and as he got further into his workout routine. The percentages would be adjusted in 8 to 12 weeks.

Sports Training Menu—Day 1

Workout starts between 6 and 10 A.M.

Have a Fruit Water before your workout

Have your meal no sooner than 45 minutes after your workout and no later than two hours after.

Breakfast 8:45 A.M. to 12:45 P.M.

5 egg whites 1 whole egg	3 protein
1 cup oatmeal	2 grains
¹/₂ raisins or choice of dried fruit (may use artificial sweetener)	1 fruit

²/₃ cup orange juice	2 fruit
16 oz. skim milk	2 milk

Lunch 11:45 A.M. to 2:45 P.M.

1 whole-wheat bagel	4 grains
3 oz. fat-free turkey	3 proteins
1 oz. provolone cheese	1 dairy
¹/₂ cup romaine lettuce/tomatoes	¹/₂ vegetable
2 cups raw vegetables	2 vegetables
¹/₂ cup fat-free French-onion dip	No substitution

Afternoon Snack 2:45 P.M. to 4:45 P.M.

1 Clif Bar	2 protein 3 grain
12 oz. V8 Splash	3 fruit
1 banana	2 fruit
8 oz. lite yogurt	1 milk
¹/₂ scoop whey protein powder	1.5 protein

Evening Meal 6 P.M. to 7 P.M.

4 oz. grilled tilapia (fish)	4 protein
¹/₂ cup wild rice	2 grain
2 cups broccoli	4 vegetables

Evening Snack 9 P.M. to 10 P.M.

1 protein shake	4.5 protein
16 oz. skim milk	2 milk

Sports Training Menu—Day 2

Workout starts between 6 and 10 A.M.

Have a Fruit Water before your workout.

Have your meal no sooner than 45 minutes after your workout and no later than two hours after.

Breakfast 8:45 A.M. to 12:45 P.M.

2 TB. natural peanut butter	2 proteins
4 slices whole-wheat toast	4 grains
16 oz. 100% cranberry juice	4 fruits
16 oz. skim milk	2 milks

Lunch 11:45 A.M. to 2:45 P.M.

2 cups whole wheat pasta	4 grains
4 oz. very lean ground beef or turkey (try to find 95% fat-free or higher)	4 proteins
1 cup marinara sauce	1 vegetables
2 cups mixed greens	2 vegetables
Limited salad dressing	1–2 fats

Afternoon Snack 2:45 P.M. to 4:45 P.M.

1 protein shake	4 proteins
Made with 8 oz. skim milk	1 milk
Add 2 cups of any choice of berries	2 fruits

Evening Meal 6 P.M. to 7 P.M.

4 oz. grilled chicken	4 proteins
½ cup whole-wheat bun	2 grains
2 cups green beans	4 vegetables
8 oz. light yogurt	1 milk
24 red grapes	2 fruits

Evening Snack 9 P.M. to 10 P.M.

1 protein shake	4.5 proteins
16 oz. skim milk	2 milks

Sports Training Menu—Day 3

Workout starts between 6 and 10 A.M.

Have a Fruit Water before your workout.

Have your meal no sooner than 45 minutes after your workout and no later than two hours after.

Breakfast 8:45 A.M. to 10 A.M.

1¹⁄₂ cup Corn Flakes	
²⁄₃ cup All-Bran	3 grains
8 oz. skim milk	1 milk
8 oz. pineapple/orange V8	2 fruit
1 protein shake	4.5 proteins

Lunch 11:45 A.M. to 2:45 P.M.

1 can Progresso or Campbell's Healthy Choice soup (lentil, fiesta, minestrone, or any bean soup)	3 grains 2 proteins
1 cup tabouli	2 grains 1 protein
2 cups carrots and celery	2 vegetables
¹⁄₂ cup fat-free dip	No substitution

Afternoon Snack 2:45 P.M. to 4:45 P.M.

1 oz. honey-roasted soy nuts or choice of nuts	2 proteins
2 whole-wheat English muffins	2 grains
2 TB. natural peanut butter	2 protein
1 navel orange	1 fruit
24 oz. skim milk	3 milks

Evening Meal 6 P.M. to 7 P.M.

4 oz. baked salmon	4 proteins
½ cup whole-wheat rice	1 grain
1½ cups broccoli spritzed with lemon	3 vegetables
2 cups mixed greens and vegetables	2 vegetables
Limited salad dressing	1–2 fats

Evening Snack 9 P.M. to 10 P.M.

1 scoop protein powder	4 proteins
16 oz. chocolate soy milk or skim milk	2 milks
½ banana	1 fruit

Supplement Suggestions:

Dawn also suggested that this athlete supplement his eating program with a high-quality multivitamin and mineral supplement, vitamin E and vitamin C, grapeseed oil, creatine, and glutamine. For more on these supplements, turn to Chapter 11 and 14.

The Least You Need to Know

- Men and women aren't much different when it comes to their basic nutritional needs. They are different in how they get their nutrition.

- Because men generally eat more than women do, their risk of developing nutrient-related problems is lower.

- Most men consume too much animal protein, which also raises fat intake. Substituting plant proteins on a regular basis will help keep fat intake in check and add other important nutrients to the diet.

- Stock up on healthy foods to keep from having to run to the convenience store when hunger pangs hit.

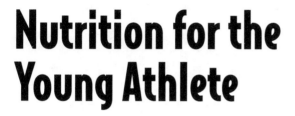

Chapter 19

Nutrition for the Young Athlete

In This Chapter

- ◆ Getting past the "ick" factor
- ◆ Necessary nutrient levels for kids and teens
- ◆ Helping kids learn how to eat right
- ◆ Kids and water

If you have children, you already know that their nutritional needs are different from yours. If your kids are active—and we're hoping that they are—making sure those nutritional needs are met will not only support their growth, it will also help them perform better on the playing field, the basketball court, the skating arena, in the pool—you name it.

It is never too soon to teach your mighty-mites some sound nutritional practices. Whether they're Little Leaguers or backyard ball bashers, get your kids eating right early on and they'll have a lifetime of good health ahead of them.

Kids vs. Food

Children of all ages are notoriously quirky and fussy about food, which can make it a real challenge for parents to ensure that their offspring eat the things they need to keep them healthy and support their growth. Young children have sensitive taste buds. For this reason, they often aren't very adventuresome about eating and it can be next to impossible to get them to try something new. Others have real aversions to specific foods. Vegetables are a classic "ick" food, but there are many others that kids will turn their noses up at and push away.

Dawn Says

If your child's idea of vegetables begins and ends with iceberg lettuce, try sneaking some nutrient-packed alternatives into his or her favorite foods. Grated zucchini and other summer squash are naturals in nut breads and muffins. You can add them to scrambled eggs, too. Nut breads and muffins can also hide grated carrots. When added to macaroni and cheese, cauliflower is almost undetectable. You might even be able to sneak in tiny broccoli florets. Spinach is usually a stretch as it's impossible to hide, but many kids don't mind it when it's mixed in with macaroni and cheese. You can also try mixing spinach into a baked potato along with some low-fat cottage cheese and a sprinkling of cheddar or Parmesan cheese for a quick stuffed potato.

Some children have such limited palates that their food choices narrow down to a few favorites. They literally eat themselves into a rut. To avoid tantrums and power struggles, parents often give into the "I won't eat it; you can't make me" syndrome and default to the foods that they know their little darlings will eat. The result is a diet that is almost guaranteed to be lacking important nutrients.

Eat It Up!

The adolescent growth spurt in girls begins at about age 10 or 11, reaches its peak at age 12, and wraps up at about age 15. Boys begin a little later—at about 12 or 13 years of age. They peak at about 14 years, but their growth spurt goes a bit longer, usually to age 19 or 20.

To add insult to injury, poor eating habits often get worse as children get older. As they approach puberty, many young people begin skipping meals. Boys and girls are both guilty of this, although girls tend to be the worst offenders, as concerns over appearance and body size begin to surface. Unfortunately, this bad habit often kicks in at about the same time that children's nutritional needs are at their highest. Puberty is a time of rapid growth, and optimal nutrition is also needed to support the hormonal changes that mark the beginning of adolescence.

When kids are active, and especially if they play sports, it is even more important to make sure that they eat right and that they know how to make good food choices on their own if you're not there to supervise them. Not only do young athletes of all shapes and sizes need more calories for energy, they also need enough of the right nutrients to support both their growth and their athletic performance.

Starting Right, Right Away

The best time to start good nutritional practices for your children is when they are very young. To ensure the best success, it's a good idea to have your own eating and exercise habits in proper order as well. Parents are not only the earliest role models that kids have when it comes to understanding what a healthy lifestyle is all about, but they are also usually the best ones. When children see their parents eating the right foods and exercising on a regular basis, they'll naturally want to follow suit. Supporting an active lifestyle for your children—even if it's just tossing a football in the backyard or driving them to and from practices and events—is another great way to drive home the message that staying fit is important.

Starting children off with good nutrition and good exercise narrows the chances of them developing bad habits that are tougher to break as they get older. As your children mature, you will have less control over their schedules and less oversight regarding what they put in their bodies. If you didn't get your kids on the right nutritional track right away, it can be a little more difficult to get them going in the right direction. However, it's not impossible and it's never too late to start.

> **Dawn Says**
>
> One of the most important habits to instill in your children early on is daily vitamin and mineral supplementation. Not everyone is in agreement on this, but the research I have read suggests that it is a good idea to reinforce nutrient intake by doing so. Very few kids get enough of the essential nutrients they need to protect their good health through the food they eat.

It can be extremely difficult to set good lifestyle examples for your kids if your own life is out of kilter. When dinner is an afterthought because you're too busy to cook, and it's slammed on the table in haste, it sends a mixed message at best and a negative message at worst. It tells your kids that food doesn't matter to you or that you don't have time to make it matter. And they'll probably extend this line of reasoning to their own behavior as they grow up.

If the meals that young people eat come out of cans and boxes or arrive at the ring of a doorbell more often than not, it will be difficult for them to see the value in home-cooked meals prepared carefully and mindfully as they grow older. Those little eyes and ears soak up everything; don't kid yourself that they don't also pick up signals when food is concerned.

Diet and exercise are issues for many parents and it can be difficult to keep these concerns in proper perspective around children. Eating disorders often begin in adolescence, but they're not unheard of in younger children. Kids who are raised in families where food serves as a pivot point for a swirl of emotional issues are especially at risk for developing their own food-related problems.

Food Foul-Ups

When food is a problem for one or both parents, it can be almost impossible to put a positive spin on it for other members of the family. However, it's vitally important that food—and exercise—be seen in a positive light. These are issues that can, and will, have a lasting impact on your children. If you're concerned that your issues with food are having a negative effect on your children, don't struggle with them on your own. Get some counseling. It might be the best thing you can do for yourself and your children.

Having young athletes in the house also necessitates teaching them how their eating choices can affect their performance. If you start this education when they are young, there will be less of a chance of their developing harmful eating habits later on.

Eat It Up!

According to a recent study, 30 to 45 percent of 9-year-old girls, and 46 to 80 percent of 10-year-old girls had already developed eating disorders.

Children who participate in sports like gymnastics, ballet and other forms of dance, wrestling, running, and figure skating are especially vulnerable to the lure of unhealthy eating, as they often feel pressure—real or imaginary—to be painfully thin in order to be competitive. These young athletes also need to understand that eating enough of the right foods is vital for optimal performance and endurance.

Beginning with the Basics

The basic diet for young athletes is based on the same sound nutritional principals that are part of any good diet. It needs to ...

- Provide sufficient calories.
- Be high in complex carbohydrates and especially nutrient-dense carbs.

- Provide a variety of different foods in each food group.

- Have a moderate amount (30 percent) of fat, saturated fat, and cholesterol.

- Contain moderate amounts of protein, sodium, salt, and sugars.

Children, like adults, need to eat throughout the day to keep their energy levels up. From the time that they're able to understand the concept of meal times, they should be coached on the importance of eating regular meals. When you're dishing out that morning oatmeal, tell them something like "Breakfast builds strong bodies." Use the analogy of the steam engine to explain why they shouldn't wait until they get tired to eat their between-meal snacks.

To ensure the best chance of getting all the nutrients young bodies need for optimum health, growth, and performance, kids also should be taught about the five essential food groups and encouraged to eat foods from all of them every day.

The USDA's food pyramid might not be the best model for adult athletes when it comes to optimal nutrition, but it works pretty well for younger sluggers. Not only that, it's colorful, and lots of food companies include it on their labeling and packaging, which makes it an ideal tool for some great on-the-spot lessons.

If there is a food pyramid on the cereal box you're pouring into that morning bowl, point it out to your kids and talk to them about it. Show them which food groups they're taking in when they eat their breakfast. Tell them what each food does for the body and talk about why it is important to eat a variety of foods from each group.

Dawn Says

Be sure to take into account the age and developmental level of your children when teaching them about nutrition. Don't get too technical when they're very young. Keep things very basic up to about when they hit grade school. By the time they're in second or third grade, they should be able to understand that dairy products like milk and yogurt help build strong bones and that eating carbohydrates like pasta, rice, potatoes, and bread gives them the energy they need for running fast and jumping high. They should also be able to understand how to visualize what proper portion sizes look like.

Nutritional Needs of Sporting Kids

As previously mentioned, active children and those who participate in sports have nutritional needs that go beyond those of children who are less active. For starters, they need more calories. In fact, they might need as much, or more, than their parents do. How much more they need largely depends on their age and how active they are. The chart below is based on the USDA food pyramid and is a good starting point for determining calorie levels and servings for children ages 6 to 12, teenage boys, and teenage girls.

Recommended Calories and Servings for Youth Athletes

	Children Ages 6 to 12 Teenage Girls	Teenage Boys
Calorie Level	About 2,200	About 2,800
Servings		
Bread Group	9	11
Vegetable Group	4	5
Fruit Group	3	4
Milk Group	2–3	2–3
Meat Group	2 (for a total of 6 ounces)	3 (for a total of 7 ounces)

As always, foods choices from the meat group should emphasize healthy, lean cuts of meat. Milk group choices should be low in fat. There are no recommended servings from the fat, oils, and sweets group at the top of the list. As a reminder, these foods add little nutritional value to the diet. As such, they should be eaten sparingly and not as a substitute for any of the foods that are lower on the nutritional pyramid.

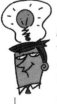

Eat It Up!

Most kids—adults, too—don't eat the minimum of five daily servings of fruits and vegetables recommended by the National Cancer Institute. Active teenagers and adolescents need even more servings than this—at least seven to nine. One possible way to get serving counts up is to have your children start the day with a serving of fruit and a glass of fruit juice. Studies show that kids who start the day with fruit are more likely to get all their servings by bedtime.

Pumping Up Calorie Counts

Depending on exercise frequency, intensity, and duration, young athletes can need as much as an extra 500 to 1,000 calories a day to meet their energy requirements. Some parents will boost calorie counts simply by serving larger portions at meals. This isn't a good idea, because it can lead to problems with portion control as kids get older. A better approach is to encourage your children to eat between-meal snacks that contain high-quality, nutrient-dense carbohydrates from the bread, fruit, milk, and vegetable groups. Possible choices include the following:

- Oatmeal-raisin cookies

- Granola bars

- Low-fat chips and crackers

- Veggies with low-fat dip

- Spaghetti

- Mini-pizzas made by topping a small pita bread with vegetables, tomato sauce, and a sprinkling of cheese

- Oatmeal with nonfat milk, fruit, and low-fat yogurt

- Homemade smoothies made with fruit, mixed with one or more of the following: low-fat yogurt or milk, silken tofu, soy milk, frozen low-fat or nonfat yogurt

- Peanut butter on whole wheat bread or low-fat whole wheat crackers

- Trail mixes. If you don't make up your own, choose products that are low in fat and sodium and don't have added sugar

- Cottage cheese and fresh fruit

- Fruit kabobs with yogurt

- Yogurt parfaits

You can make it convenient for your kids to get the extra calories they need by stocking healthy snack choices in your pantry. Stick take-along snacks in their backpacks for after-school practice sessions or away games. Give them boxes of granola or energy bars to store in their lockers at school. The easier you make it for them to make healthy choices, the less likely they'll be to grab for high-fat, high-sugar foods from school vending machines or fast-food restaurants when hunger overtakes them.

If your kids are finicky eaters, it might be tough to get them to choose healthy food to augment their calorie intake. While high-quality carbs are always going to deliver the best nutritional bang per calorie, it's okay to let young athletes have some simple carbohydrates to boost their nutrient intake once in a while. An occasional soft drink or candy bar will not only help supply part of their calorie needs, it will keep kids from feeling deprived, especially when their friends are enjoying these treats.

You can tell if your child is eating enough calories by tracking his or her height and weight. If he or she is gaining weight, but not height, it might be time to cut back on the serving sizes of snacks, or substitute some lower-calorie alternatives. Don't eliminate them completely, and never cut back on the food choices at main meals. It's important to get your kids into the habit of eating enough food for these meals, as doing so will help them eat right as adults.

Your child's athletic performance is another good gauge of adequate nutrient intake. If he or she is doing well both while competing or working out and afterward, then it's a good indication that he or she is eating right. However, if he or she is feeling fatigued, draggy, or irritable, then he or she probably needs more to eat and probably more to drink as well. We'll discuss hydration needs of young athletes later in this chapter.

As discussed in Chapter 17, young female athletes, especially those who are highly competitive in physically challenging sports, also run the risk of developing serious long-term health problems if they don't take in enough food to meet their energy needs. It's important to keep an eye on what your kids eat regardless of the reason, but especially so when it comes to children in this at-risk population. Your good counsel might cause some temper tantrums, especially if your daughter is feeling pressured into maintaining a low body weight in order to compete at top form, but any fights that may erupt are well worth the long-term benefits of such intervention.

More About Kids and Carbohydrates

Young athletes need carbohydrates to fuel their performance just like adults do. They need to eat enough carbs on a regular basis, and especially after exercise, to keep their glycogen levels where they should be for optimal performance.

Like adults, many young athletes tend to take in more protein than they really need, which means their carbohydrate levels are lower than they should be. Active children should eat 50 to 55 percent of their total calories as carbohydrates, or about 2.7 grams of carbohydrates per pound of body weight. As an example, if your young athlete weighs 120 pounds, he or she would need to eat around 324 grams of carbohydrates per day.

To meet their carbohydrate needs, encourage your kids to eat complex carbohydrates—vegetables, whole-grain breads, pasta, cereals, brown rice, and so on—instead of the simple carbohydrates contained in milk and fruit. Choosing complex carbohydrates will also give them better supplies of some essential nutrients, such as B vitamins, iron, dietary fiber, and other important vitamins and minerals.

Kids and Protein

All kids need protein in order to grow well and build strong muscles. If they eat balanced meals, most children get enough protein in their diets. However, adequate protein intake can be a problem for athletic children. Active kids need between 0.5 to 1 gram of protein daily per pound of body weight, depending on activity level. This equates to 50 to 100 grams of protein for a child who weighs 100 pounds. Hitting the mark for dairy intake can provide most of the protein that young athletes need. Small servings of protein at lunch and dinner should get levels to where they need to be.

Kids who don't drink much milk are at a greater risk for protein deficiency. If you have young ones at home who don't care for the white stuff, try them on other dairy products like yogurt and low-fat cheeses. Another way to boost dairy intake is to add powdered milk to baked goods and smoothies. Doing so will increase both protein and calcium intake. Although it's not a good idea to give kids too much fruit juice, some juices are now calcium fortified.

Kids and Fat

All of the warnings about fat that have surfaced in recent years are directed mostly at adults, but we tend to forget that they are. As a result, adults sometimes get a little overzealous when it comes to restricting fat intake for their kids. While it's important for everyone to keep a close eye on how much fat they eat, and to keep levels within reason, growing bodies can tolerate a little more fat intake—in fact, children generally need to get about 30 percent of their calories from fat for optimum nutrition. When kids eat diets that are too low in fat, they run the risk of not taking in enough energy.

The Right Stuff at the Right Times

When young athletes eat is just as important as what they eat. As is the case with adult athletes, timing is everything when it comes to fueling performance.

Dawn Says
Give your child too much to eat too close to a training session or game and it might slow him or her down instead of boost him or her up. The closer you get to game time, the smaller meals need to be. As a general rule, it's wise to allow three to four hours for a large meal to digest, two to three hours for a small meal, one to two hours for a liquid meal (such as a smoothie), and less than one hour for a small meal or snack. As you get closer to the event, food choices should emphasize complex carbohydrates and be very low in protein and fat.

Beating the Breakfast Blues

Breakfast, of course, is the most important meal of the day for children as well as adults. The energy your kids need for their afternoon practice sessions and competitions begins with this all-important meal. When they skip it, they start the day with an energy deficit and it can be tough for them to make up that deficit by the time they hit the playing field.

Like adults, many young people find it difficult to eat breakfast. Some don't care for traditional breakfast foods. Other kids aren't very hungry when they wake up. If they're in a rush to get to school, or they have early morning practices, eating might be the last thing on their minds. For these reasons and others, a lot of kids skip breakfast entirely or wait until later in the morning to eat it when they finally get hungry. Both habits are bad ones to get into and bad ones for parents to indulge.

A better approach is to think outside the box a little when it comes to breakfast entrées. If your kids don't like cereal, experiment with some other foods until you find ones that will tickle the taste buds in the morning. Lots of kids might turn up their noses at cereal and fruit, but they'll eat leftover spaghetti or macaroni and cheese. These dishes can be just as healthy as traditional breakfast entrées if they're prepared right to begin with.

Other substitutes for traditional breakfasts include the following:

- Peanut butter on low-fat, whole-wheat crackers

- Rice pudding

- Baked potatoes

- Low-fat, low-sodium pizza or lasagna

- Milk shakes made with low-fat or nonfat milk, low-fat ice cream or yogurt, tofu, and fruit

- Breakfast bars

- Breakfast burritos made with whole-wheat or corn tortillas, tofu or beans, and salsa

- Yogurt parfaits, made with low-fat yogurt and fruit and topped with a sprinkling of nuts or cereal

The goal is to get your kids to eat a high-carb breakfast and to do so on a regular basis. If it has to come by way of breakfast bar, or even an ice-cream-based shake, so be it. Anything—yes, this is true—is better than nothing.

Pregame Nutrition Strategies

Eating a healthy meal before a game or practice is important for maintaining energy levels both during the activity and after it. Making sure your kids eat right before a game is fairly easy if you can sit them down for a pregame meal at home, but this often isn't possible. When young athletes travel to a meet or an away game and you can't be with them, they might be on their own when it comes to making sure they get what they need before competition.

One of the best ways to ensure proper nutrition when you can't be there to provide it is to map out a pregame eating strategy with your kids. Go through their training and competition schedules and determine what they should be eating and drinking as well as when. To make sure they get what they need, load a backpack or athletic bag with take-along foods like snack bars, bagels, fruit, fruit or vegetable juice, sandwiches, and so on, that they can take with them.

The biggest thing to remember is that less is more when you get closer to the event. Also, pre-event food choices must emphasize carbohydrates and be lower in fat and protein. Peanut butter is a bad choice right before a game as it's hard to digest, but three to four hours afterward it's a great choice for helping muscles recover from exertion. The best way to find out what works for your young athletes is through experimentation. Make sure to limit your experiments to practices, though. The day of the big game is not the time to be trying new foods that may not be tolerated well. For more information on pregame and postgame eating for kids, turn to Appendix B.

> **Dawn Says**
>
> Try to have a variety of snacks. The food bag concept is great! You spend time packing the proper clothes and equipment—why not their food?

If you're transporting your kids to their practices and games, you can use the same strategy to help you plan ahead so you can have healthy foods and beverages in the car for them to eat on the way and back.

Postgame Eating

Postgame eating is important as well to replenish the glycogen levels in the muscles and liver. Try to get your kids to eat a carbohydrate snack within 30 minutes after their activity. This snack should contain between 15 to 30 grams of carbs—the amount found in the following snacks:

- A glass of milk and a piece of fruit
- A 12–16 ounce smoothie

- Two ounces of mini-bagels
- A yogurt cup and a piece of fruit

Follow this up with a well-balanced meal within two hours of the practice or event.

If there is a victory to celebrate, chances are pretty good that the festivities will take place at a fast-food spot or other restaurant where good nutritional choices are limited. If this is the case, you've got two options: Let the kids have what they want—within reason, of course—or try to steer them to the healthiest things on the menu. If you can keep them from supersizing their selections, having a celebratory burger, fries, and shake isn't out of the question. Encouraging your kids to stick to the simplest items on the menu—for example, a plain cheeseburger, or a grilled chicken breast sandwich—is another positive approach to fast-food eating.

Water Woes

Active children also have special fluid needs that have to be met. Like adults, they need to drink before, during, and after practice sessions or competition and they need to do so whether they feel thirsty or not. Another key piece of nutritional education that parents are responsible for is stressing to their young athletes the importance of staying hydrated and stressing what good hydration does for performance.

Kids, like adults, tend to go by their feelings of thirst to determine when they should drink water. However, by the time the "I'm thirsty" signal kicks in, their bodies are already dehydrated.

> ### Dawn Says
>
> Children who participate in water sports or cold-weather sports need to drink just as much water as do other young athletes. However, they often don't sense the need as easily as the others do because they aren't as aware of the fluids they lose through sweating. It's especially important to make sure that the kids who participate in these sports learn how to drink on a schedule and that they take water bottles with them to facilitate doing so.

If your young athlete gets tired easily at practice or fades during competition, dehydration might be the culprit. Other indications of low hydration levels in children include these:

- Crankiness or irritability
- Dark- or bright-colored urine that has a strong odor

- ◆ Sunken eyes

- ◆ Dry tongue and lips

- ◆ Infrequent urination

- ◆ Reduced urine volume

Dehydration is dangerous for children and adults alike, but it can be especially so for young athletes. Because kids don't cool off as efficiently as adults do, they overheat and become dehydrated more easily, which puts them at greater risk for developing heat exhaustion or heatstroke. In a young child, losing a half-pound of weight through sweat can cause a significant decrease in performance. Teenagers need just as much water as adults do—at least eight 8-ounce glasses of the clear stuff a day. Younger athletes should drink between five and eight 8-ounce glasses a day. Before strenuous activity, children should drink 4 to 8 ounces of fluids. During activity, fluid intake should be at least 4 ounces of fluids for every 15 minutes. Teenagers need to up their intake to 6 to 8 ounces every 15 to 20 minutes.

> **Dawn Says**
>
> Make it easy for your kids to drink their water by giving them each their own water bottle. Make it fun for little kids to tell how much they drink by buying bottles that have marks to indicate ounces or milliliters.

If there are times when your child isn't thrilled about drinking water, sports drinks are a good substitute. They're definitely more expensive than water, but kids often find them more appealing than plain water because they taste better. Sports drinks also stimulate thirst, which means your kids will end up drinking more fluids.

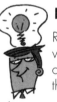

> **Eat It Up!**
>
> Research shows that kids will drink 90 percent more of a flavored sports drink than water.

Sports drinks are absorbed just as quickly as water. They're a good source of carbohydrates for working muscles during exercise and especially for workouts or practices that last an hour or more. They're also good for days when more than one workout or exercise period is scheduled.

The best sports drink selections are those that contain between 4 to 8 percent carbohydrate. Anything more than this can delay fluid absorption when kids need it most. Kids are big fans of carbonated drinks. It's okay to let them have a soft drink now and again, but they need to understand that moderation is important when it comes to carbonated or sugary beverages, because they can interfere with training and competition schedules. These drinks are absorbed slowly and they contain high-fructose corn syrup, which can cause stomach cramps, nausea, and diarrhea. Water, as always, is the best beverage choice for pint-sized athletes and adults alike.

The Least You Need to Know

◆ Young athletes need more calories than their more sedentary counterparts. When adding calories to the diet, it's best to give kids nutrient-dense between-meal snacks instead of increasing main-meal portion sizes.

◆ Eating regularly is always key to athletic performance. Make sure your kids don't skip meals. Encourage them to eat regularly throughout the day so they'll have a consistent source of energy to fuel their activities.

◆ It's okay to let your children have an occasional sweet treat or soft drink. However, they should only be eaten in addition to, not in place of, more nutritious foods from other food groups.

◆ If your young athletes eat the number of servings recommended on the food pyramid, they should be able to get the vitamins, minerals, and calories they need. However, most children don't eat a balanced diet on a regular basis. A good daily multivitamin/multimineral supplement guarantees adequate nutrient levels for all children—and adults, too.

Chapter 20

Nutrition for the Senior Athlete

In This Chapter

- The special nutritional needs of older athletes
- The role of exercise in battling disease and physical decline
- Senior hydration needs
- Supplements for seniors

It used to be that the golden years meant kicking back in a rocking chair and taking it easy. Not anymore. Today's seniors are more active than any of their age group in prior generations. They're reaping the benefits of a healthy lifestyle, and are using that good health to propel their longevity.

Sports are no longer just a young person's arena, either. Seniors are competing in endurance events like marathons and triathlons in greater numbers than ever before. There may be no real "fountain of youth," but seniors are finding the next best thing to it through good nutrition and exercise.

The Shape of Senior Athletes

Like athletes of all ages, senior athletes come in all shapes and sizes. Some were active and athletic when they were young and have continued their healthy lifestyles as they've aged. Others may not have actively embraced exercise when they were young, but are taking to it as they get older.

Research has shown that exercise can do all sorts of wonderful things for people in the later stages of life. Among its many benefits, staying active can …

- Fight declines in flexibility, strength, muscle mass, and aerobic capacity.

- Reduce risk factors related to heart disease, high blood pressure, osteoporosis, and type-II diabetes.

- Help ward off "middle age spread"—the creeping levels of body fat that tend to increase with age.

- Improve balance and help prevent injuries from falling.

- Improve immune function.

- Cope better with stress.

- Improve body composition—that is, reduce body fat levels while increasing lean tissue levels.

Eat It Up!

According to USA Triathlon, the number of triathlon participants who can also claim membership to AARP is twice that of athletes in their late teens. Triathletes in their 40s substantially out number those in their 20s.

Eat It Up!

According to researchers, the combination of a nutrient-rich diet and physical activity can protect seniors from a number of age-related degenerative diseases as well as other mental and physical declines related to aging, including diminished mental function, decreased physical function, weight loss, social withdrawal, and malnutrition.

Over the past few years, researchers have found that seniors of all fitness levels can respond to strength and endurance training nearly just as well as their younger counterparts do. Both older men and older women who participated in various studies gained in strength and cardiovascular capacity. It might take them a little longer to see results, but if they stick with their programs, they will. Obviously, it's never too late when it comes to reaping the benefits of exercising and eating properly.

Staying active is clearly a key to enjoying a long life and staying healthy while you do so. For seniors, following an eating plan that matches their intake to activities and energy output will ensure that they'll have enough energy to get the most out of what they do and keep their weight at healthy levels.

In the coming years, you'll see a greater emphasis on research that addresses many issues related to aging—including exercise and nutrition—as the baby-boom generation grows older. It's estimated that by the year 2010, 1 in 5 people in the United States will be 65 or older, compared to 1 in 10 in 1980. As lifetimes continue to get longer, it will be even more important to find ways to help seniors stay healthy and independent.

Senior Nutritional Issues

Seniors have some age-related nutritional issues that are both caused by decreased activity levels and that affect their ability to stay active. For starters, as people get older, their basal metabolic rate (BMR) slows down unless they maintain activity levels equal to or slightly more than what they did when they were in their 30s. A lower BMR decreases their energy requirements, which means they have to eat less to maintain an optimal weight. As calorie needs decrease, it can be difficult for seniors to get enough nutrients from the foods they eat.

> **Eat It Up!**
>
> According to researchers, it's a good idea for seniors to increase their activity levels as they get older, or to modestly reduce their calorie intake while making more nutritious food choices. Keeping energy output at a constant level throughout the middle-age years doesn't prevent adults from having to deal with "middle-age spread." In one study, men who maintained a constant weekly running distance through middle age put on 3.3 pounds and gained ³/₄ inch in waist circumference per decade. It didn't matter what distance they ran; they all gained weight. Although researchers don't know the exact reason for the gain, they believe it's related to declines in testosterone and growth hormone.

Older bodies also process food differently. It's estimated that as many as 30 percent of seniors over age 65 develop something called *atrophic gastritis*, which means they can no longer produce enough stomach acid to be able to digest certain vitamins and minerals, such as vitamin B12, folic acid, calcium, and iron. This problem gets worse as people get older. By age 80, as many as 40 percent of seniors aren't able to absorb some important nutrients due to decreased stomach acid levels.

Many seniors suffer from nutritional deficiencies caused by lower calorie intake, poor menu planning, chronic diseases, interactions between

> **Foodie**
>
> **Atrophic gastritis** is the inability to produce stomach acid.

drugs and nutrients, malabsorption, and, sadly, malnutrition, which is a particular problem for older people who are on low-fixed incomes. The nutritional deficiencies most often seen are the following:

- Vitamin A, leading to vision problems, dry skin, and lower immunity levels. Taking in too much vitamin A, however, can also cause problems because it won't leave the system as quickly as it does in younger people.

- Vitamin B1 (thiamin), believed to be very common among seniors. Supple-mental thiamin has been shown to improve energy levels, sleep, and general quality of life.

- Vitamin B6. Reduced absorption of this nutrient leads to increased risk of heart disease and other disorders.

- Folic acid. Reduced levels play a role in the development of cardiovascular disease and may also cause or worsen brain function problems. Folic acid also protects against stroke and cancer.

- Vitamin B12. An estimated 12 to 14 percent of seniors are believed to be deficient in vitamin B12 due to their inability to absorb it. Low B12 levels also contribute to impaired mental capacity, cognitive dysfunction, and other central nervous system disorders. Low B12 levels can also reduce immunity.

Eat It Up!

Vitamin D deficiency has been shown to worsen the symptoms of osteoarthritis, such as cartilage breakdown and the development of bony spurs called osteophytes. In one study, researchers found a three-times-greater risk of osteoarthritis progressing in seniors who didn't take in enough vitamin D. However, there was no evidence that low levels of vitamin D would cause osteoarthritis in normal joints.

- Vitamin D. Seniors often lack this important vitamin for three reasons: their ability to absorb it decreases with age, they often get less sun, and they are less able to synthesize it in their skin. This deficiency increases the risk for osteoporosis, diabetes, arthritis, and some cancers.

- Calcium. Seniors both eat fewer foods that contain calcium and absorb less of it. Combined with vitamin D deficiency, calcium deficiency contributes to decreased bone densities, resulting in fractures. Low calcium levels also contribute to hypertension and colon cancer.

- Iron. Low levels of this important micronutrient result from not eating enough calories or protein, combined with impaired iron absorption.

- Magnesium. Magnesium assists protein metabolism and is also important for muscle contraction and nerve impulse transmission. People over age 55, however, are at increased risk for experiencing side effects such as appetite loss, diarrhea, irregular heartbeat, and abdominal pain if they take in too much magnesium, which is also found in certain antacids.

◆ Zinc. Zinc is important for wound healing in all individuals. In older people, it may also support immune function, although some studies contradict this.

Supplementation ensures adequate amounts of these nutrients in all people. Seniors, due to their impaired ability to absorb many nutrients, need higher doses of many of these nutrients. For example, seniors over 70 need three times the amount of vitamin D—600 IU—than people under 50.

Smell and Taste Issues

As people age, they lose their ability to taste and smell. This happens for a variety of reasons. It's partially due to the aging process itself, but it can also be caused by certain medications, disease, and injury. Not being able to taste or smell food doesn't make it much fun to eat, which is why many seniors suffer from poor nutrition. Researchers are exploring ways to make food more palatable for seniors by adding odor and flavor enhancers.

Special Hydration Needs

The amount of water the body contains gradually declines as people age, which means they're at greater risk of becoming dehydrated unless they keep their water consumption up. The problem is, older people also don't feel thirsty as much or as frequently as younger people do. Some older people even avoid water because of concerns over urinary incontinence. This leads to a number of health problems, including impaired kidney function.

When seniors are active, they run an even higher risk of becoming dehydrated, especially if their activities take place in hot, humid weather.

The Senior Food Pyramid

The average senior needs to take in anywhere from 1,200 to approximately 1,600 calories a day just to support his or her basic activities. Men, of course, will need more calories than women, but these levels seem to be about right for most seniors. They reflect the following number of servings recommended by the food guide pyramid:

- Three servings from the milk, yogurt, and cheese group

- Two servings from the meat, poultry, fish, dry beans, eggs, and nut group

- Two to three servings from the vegetable group

- Two servings from the fruit group

- Six servings from the bread, fortified cereal, rice, and pasta group

The Tufts University USDA Human Nutrition Research Center on Aging has even developed a food pyramid for seniors 70 and older that reflect these intake levels. It's similar to the standard food guide pyramid in most respects, but it makes several important recommendations that the standard pyramid does not make. As a reflection of older adults' lower hydration and thirst levels, it recommends drinking eight 8-ounce glasses of water every day.

> **Dawn Says**
>
> If you find it difficult to drink enough water to meet your daily liquid requirements, you can substitute juice, milk, sports drinks, and noncaffeinated soft drinks and beverages. These items can count as 50 percent of your daily requirement for liquid.

The senior food guide pyramid also recommends supplementing the diet with additional calcium, vitamin D, and vitamin B12—the vitamins that older adults can't absorb and process as well. Finally, the senior food guide pyramid emphasizes fiber intake in the form of whole grains, legumes, and whole fruits and vegetables. Fiber not only helps prevent constipation and hemorrhoids by assisting the transit of waste through the intestines, it can help lower cholesterol levels and reduce the risk of heart disease and cancer. Twenty to thirty grams of fiber is recommended daily for optimal health.

Special Nutritional Needs for Active Seniors

Older adults who stay active on a regular basis can usually eat more because their energy needs are higher. What's more, they don't need to be knocking themselves out doing high-energy aerobics or training for marathons to boost calorie needs. Activities such as yoga, dancing, swimming, playing golf, walking, and resistance training can also increase calorie consumption. The key is exercising on a regular basis, not just in spurts for short periods of time.

If it's necessary to decrease calories because of weight gain, it's even more important to select foods that are rich in nutrients to offset the decrease in nutrient absorption that comes along with aging.

Eat It Up!

Seniors surveyed at the 1999 National Senior Game–Senior Olympics said that exercise was the biggest factor in their being able to lead an active lifestyle. Other key contributors identified by the seniors were, in order, lifestyle in general, diet, genetics, and work. Even though 64 percent of the seniors participating in the games reported having to take prescription medication to treat an age-related condition, 90 percent of them said they felt they were in much better or somewhat better health than other people their own age. While seniors said their health and personal pride meant more to them than winning, 71 percent also said that they felt their sport kept them healthy.

Choosing whole foods over refined products as much as possible is an easy way to increase vitamin and mineral intake. Other nutrient-boosting habits to get into include eating raw vegetables and fruit at least once a day, and cooking vegetables as little as possible, since prolonged soaking and boiling leaches vitamins, especially B1 and C, from food.

Protein and Seniors

Experts used to think that the decrease in lean body mass that happens as people get older was related to inadequate protein intake. We now know that decreases in lean body mass are related to lower activity levels, not lack of protein. Increasing lean body mass through exercise will enable the body to use protein to make muscle instead of fat.

Cashing In on Calcium

Adequate calcium intake, coupled with exercise, is the best way to fight osteoporosis and slow down its progress. Getting enough calcium is also important for defending against hypertension and colon cancer; however, older people don't absorb calcium well due to decreases in stomach acid production.

In addition, calcium intake among older individuals is often low because they don't like the taste of milk or they can't digest it due to lactose intolerance. Because of this, many of them depend on calcium supplements to boost their levels of this important nutrient. However, the calcium in supplements is often poorly absorbed. Other ways to boost calcium intake include:

◆ Experimenting with other dairy products. Products such as yogurt and cheese may not cause the same digestion problems as milk does.

- Adding powdered milk to baked goods.

- Using yogurt as a base for salad dressings and dips.

- Eating dark leafy greens, which are a good source of calcium.

- Eating sardines and other fish with edible bones.

- Eating nuts and seeds that are rich in calcium, such as almonds, brazils, macadamias, pecans, pistachios, sesame seeds, and sunflower seeds.

Some types of orange and vegetable juice are now calcium enriched. Tofu made with calcium sulphate is another good source of calcium as well as protein.

Increasing Iron

Red meat and organ meats are always the best sources of dietary iron because the body better absorbs the form of iron found in these foods. Iron from plant sources can be better absorbed if they're eaten along with a small amount of animal protein, or with something that's rich in vitamin C—such as fruit juice or raw or lightly cooked vegetables—at the same time.

Fluid Facts

Staying active increases the need for fluids beyond the recommended 64 ounces a day. Good hydration levels are especially important for seniors who participate in competitive sports like running, tennis, cycling, and golf, where weather conditions and activity duration can substantially affect hydration levels. Because thirst sensitivity decreases with age, seniors need to establish a drinking schedule and not depend on their thirst levels to signal a water stop.

When exercising, seniors should drink small amounts of fluids on a regular basis. A good rule of thumb is about 4 ounces of water every 15 minutes. Drinking a cup of water—8 ounces—an hour before working out, and chasing it with another 4 to 8 ounces of water 15 minutes before exertion, will also help keep hydration levels where they should be.

Seniors who compete in athletic events need to be even more careful about starting out with good hydration levels and maintaining them. Important hydration strategies for this group include:

- Monitoring water intake for several days before an event and increasing fluid intake if necessary. One of the best ways to gauge adequate hydration is to check urine color—the paler, the better.

◆ Avoiding alcohol (a proven dehydrator) for at least 24 hours before an event.

◆ Using sports drinks when necessary to assist rehydration. Experiment with a couple of them well in advance of the competition to determine which ones work best.

If water loss is a particular concern, seniors should weigh themselves immediately before and after competing to gauge how much water they've lost. For every pound of weight lost, drink 3 cups (24 ounces) of fluid.

For more information on proper hydration before and after working out or competing, turn to Chapter 3.

Supplements for Seniors

The combination of absorption problems and diets that lack important nutrients makes vitamin and mineral supplementation a necessity for all seniors. Taking a quality multi-vitamin/multimineral daily is a good start. Taking supplements that are formulated as antioxidants is even better. As previously discussed, seniors often need additional levels of certain nutrients, including the B vitamins, calcium, and iron, that go beyond what even the best multivitamins contain. Getting enough of them means taking additional supplements.

Creatine, a popular supplement for young athletes looking for ways to improve their competitive edge, may also give older exercisers a needed boost. Recent research found that older men who took the supplement increased in strength in as little as a week. Other studies have shown that creatine may play a positive role in combating a number of neuromuscular diseases, such as Parkinson's disease, muscular dystrophy, and other muscle-wasting disorders.

Other supplements that may be of benefit to seniors include:

◆ Fish oil. A good source of heart-healthy omega-3 oils, fish oil has also been shown to be beneficial for maintaining joint health and in relieving arthritis symptoms.

◆ Glucosamine sulfate. A number of studies have shown that this supplement can reduce joint pain and improve range of motion in people with osteoarthritis.

◆ Garlic. Some research supports garlic's ability to reduce stroke risks by lowering cholesterol and blood pressure.

Although it's always a good idea to let your physician know about any supplements that you're taking, it's especially important for seniors to discuss their supplement use with their primary care physicians. Some popular supplements can negatively impact the effects of various drugs—ginkgo biloba, for example, has blood-thinning properties and shouldn't be taken by anyone using anticoagulant medications—and can seriously affect senior health.

The Least You Need to Know

◆ Being active is important for enjoying a long life and good health.

◆ Seniors need to follow an eating plan that matches their intake to their activities and energy output to ensure they have enough energy.

◆ Because thirst sensitivity decreases with age, seniors need to follow a schedule for taking in fluids when they're active.

◆ Most seniors need additional vitamin and mineral supplementation to make up for what they can't absorb from the food they eat.

Chapter 21

The Vegetarian Athlete

In This Chapter

- Defining the vegetarian
- The benefits of vegetarian eating
- Learning how to eat veggie style
- Understanding soy products

Eat less meat, eat more veggies. We've all heard this mantra repeated pretty regularly in recent years. More and more people are jumping on the vegetarian bandwagon for a variety of reasons—their good health being just one of them. But can a diet that includes no animal protein, or very small amounts, be good for athletes with special nutritional needs? Absolutely! The good news is that by paying extra attention to getting some important nutrients, a vegetarian diet can be healthy for everyone.

Besides being perfectly healthy for athletes to be vegetarians, there is even evidence that eating a vegetarian diet can boost your energy better than one that emphasizes meat as a protein source. When you're going for the competitive edge, eating vegetarian style might be just the secret weapon you're looking for.

What Is a Vegetarian?

A vegetarian is typically defined as someone who doesn't eat meat. But this is just a basic definition. Within the vegetarian world there are various versions of "not eating meat." As detailed on the following chart, all vegetarians avoid meat and meat products. Some will eat dairy products, others eschew anything derived from animals or their slaughter. They won't eat meat, wear leather products, or use cosmetics and other products that contain ingredients that come from animals.

Types of Vegetarians

Lacto-Ovo Vegetarian	The most common type of vegetarian in Western cultures Avoids meat, fish, poultry, and most foods derived from animal slaughter Will eat dairy products, eggs, and honey
Lacto Vegetarian	Avoids meat, fish, poultry, and most foods derived from animal slaughter Avoids eggs and foods made with eggs Will eat dairy products and usually honey
Ovo Vegetarian	Avoids meat, fish, poultry, and most foods derived from animal slaughter Avoids dairy products and foods made from these products Will eat eggs and usually honey
Vegan	Avoids all foods containing animal products including meat, fish, poultry, eggs, dairy, and often honey Often will not wear leather, wool, or silk, or use cosmetics and household products containing animal ingredients or byproducts Many also avoid sugar as some sugar is filtered through activated charcoal that may be derived from animal bones
Pescetarian	Avoids meat and poultry Will eat fish, eggs, and dairy Some will eat free-range meat and poultry
Fruitarian	Eats only fruits and certain vegetables that are technically fruit, such as tomatoes, cucumbers, squash, and avocados Will also eat nuts and seeds

There are three additional types of vegetarianism that can be considered subsets of the main groups:

♦ Macrobiotics. This dietary philosophy has its roots in Eastern cultures. It advocates eating seasonal foods, which are prepared and consumed based on the yin and yang principles of balance and harmony. The diet varies somewhat according to the specific macrobiotic tradition being followed (there are several). Foods from the nightshade family, such as potatoes, eggplant, peppers, etc., are not eaten.

♦ Raw foods. Individuals who follow the raw foods philosophy eat—you guessed it—only foods in their raw state, including vegetables, fruits, nuts, seeds, sprouted grains, and legumes.

♦ Raw living foods, or living foods. Similar to raw foods, people who follow this dietary philosophy warm up some of their food but stop short of cooking them at high temperatures in order to preserve the enzymes contained in raw foods.

♦ Natural hygiene. This dietary philosophy promotes the consumption of foods that are unadulterated and in their natural state, such as fruits, vegetables, nuts, seeds, sprouted grains, and legumes. Limited amounts of animal products are sometimes added. Foods are eaten in specific combinations believed to be best for efficient digestion.

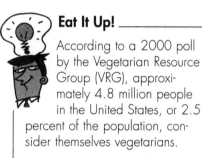

Eat It Up!

According to a 2000 poll by the Vegetarian Resource Group (VRG), approximately 4.8 million people in the United States, or 2.5 percent of the population, consider themselves vegetarians.

As you can see, there are many variations on the vegetarian lifestyle. Some people who occasionally eat animal protein also consider themselves vegetarians as they follow a vegetarian diet more often than not.

Why People Go Vegetarian

Eating a diet that's rich in whole grains, fruits, and vegetables is simply a lot healthier than one that's heavy in protein and saturated fat. The health benefits of vegetarianism are the main appeal of this way of eating, but it's not the only reason more people are embracing it. Some choose to for religious reasons. Others support the ecological, economic, and ethical facets of vegetarianism. Going vegetarian helps conserve fossil fuels and water, as it takes less of both commodities to produce plant foods as opposed to animal protein. In fact, it takes 3 to 15 times more water to keep animals hydrated than it does to produce plant crops.

The Vegetarian Athlete

Many athletes have embraced vegetarianism as their preferred way of eating. Among them are world-class and Olympic champions in many sports in all categories, including strength, speed, and endurance. They include the following:

◆ Billie Jean King, tennis

◆ Martina Navratilova, tennis

◆ Hank Aaron, baseball

◆ Surya Bonaly, champion figure skater

◆ Walter "Killer" Kowalski, pro wrestler

◆ Andreas Cahling, pro bodybuilder, IFBB Mr. International

◆ Edwin Moses, track and field, Olympic gold medalist in the 400m hurdles

◆ Paavo Nurmi, Olympic champion middle- and long-distance runner

◆ Rob Sweetgall, world champion ultra-distance racewalker

◆ Murray Rose, swimmer, four-time Olympic gold medalist

◆ Bill Walton, basketball

◆ Bill Manetti, powerlifting champion

◆ Bill Pearl, bodybuilder, four-time "Mr. Universe"

You just have to believe that vegetarianism works when you see burly powerlifters who swear by their vegetarian diets lifting hundreds of pounds above their heads without a second thought. However, vegetarianism has received somewhat of a bad rap in the sporting world in the past, mostly due to misconceptions about what a vegetarian diet is all about. Until recently, it was widely believed that vegetarianism:

◆ Could not provide enough calories to fuel optimum performance.

◆ Could not provide enough protein to support optimal cell growth and regeneration.

◆ Required combining various carbohydrates at each meal to create complete protein—the "complementary protein" theory.

◆ Could not provide adequate levels of certain micronutrients, such as calcium, iron, B12, and zinc.

Eat It Up!

The complementary protein theory in vegetarianism relates to the fact that plant proteins are incomplete because they lack one or more of the essential amino acids or have low levels of them. Until fairly recently it was believed that you had to eat certain combinations of plant foods—beans and rice, for example, or peanut butter and whole-wheat bread—during the same meal to get the same nutritional benefit that animal-based protein delivers. More recent research, however, doesn't support this theory. As long as you eat a good variety of plant proteins during the course of the day, you'll get all the complete protein you need.

Nutritional researchers have taken a hard look at many of the concerns surrounding vegetarianism and athletic performance and have proven most of them wrong. Their research supports the fact that a vegetarian diet can provide adequate protein if enough calories are consumed and if it contains a variety of plant proteins such as legumes, grains, nuts, and seeds. And there is no need to eat complementary proteins at each meal as long as a variety of plant proteins are eaten during the course of a day.

However, this isn't to say that there aren't some concerns related to vegetarianism. People who choose to eat a vegetarian diet do need to be careful about picking foods that will supply sufficient amounts of the micronutrients listed here:

◆ Iron. All athletes, and especially women who participate in endurance events, run the risk of being low in iron. This can be a particular problem when following a vegetarian diet, as your body won't absorb the iron in plant foods (non-heme iron) as well as it does in animal foods (heme iron). This doesn't mean you should switch back to eating animal protein. What it does mean is that you'll have to eat a lot of iron-rich plant foods. Choices include spinach, chard, dried beans, blackstrap molasses, dried fruits, and bulgur wheat. Some breakfast cereals are also fortified with iron.

◆ Calcium. Calcium is present in plant foods, but at a lower level than in animal protein. If you choose plant foods with good levels of calcium, you should be able to meet your daily calcium requirements with no problems. Food choices here include broccoli, kale, collard greens,

Dawn Says

Iron absorption can also be affected if you drink tea or coffee with your meals. A better choice is orange juice, which will boost the amount of iron absorbed. If you're going to drink tea or coffee, do so at least an hour or two before or after you eat. Cooking your foods in cast iron cookware, which leaches absorbable iron into food, is another easy way to boost iron intake.

beans, bok choy, tahini, turnip greens, and calcium-fortified orange juice, grains, and soy products. If you're a lacto-ovo vegetarian—the most common type—you won't have to worry about calcium as much because you'll get it in dairy products.

◆ B12. Animal foods are the primary source for this vitamin, so if you're eating some animal protein you won't have to worry as much about it. Getting enough B12, however, is a problem for strict vegetarians and especially for vegans. You can get B12 in foods that are fortified with it, such as some breads, cereals, soy products, and nutritional yeast. Not all of these products contain B12, so be sure to read labels carefully. You can also take a B12 supplement. Choose one that provides 100 percent of the RDA.

◆ Riboflavin. Another potential problem for strict vegetarians and vegans, as animal protein is also a leading source for riboflavin. Plant sources include whole-grain cereal, dark green leafy vegetables, mushrooms, sweet potatoes, soybeans, avocados, nuts, and sea vegetables. If you're eating dairy products, you should be okay.

◆ Creatine. The jury is still out on whether this supplement has all the performance-boosting abilities that some say it does, but research does show that it can improve performance for athletes who compete in sports that require quick, short bursts of energy. However, it is another micronutrient that can be difficult to get enough of in a vegetarian diet. For this reason, you might want to take a second look at it.

◆ Zinc. Again, more of a concern for strict vegetarians than those who eat some animal protein. Zinc is found in plant foods, but it's in a form that makes it more difficult to be absorbed than that found in animal protein. Studies have shown zinc supplementation to have no benefit on athletic performance, so you're better off eating foods that contain it, including whole-grain products, wheat germ, legumes, nuts, tofu, hard cheeses, and fortified cereals.

Food Foul-Ups

A vegetarian diet does not mean eating french fries and milkshakes instead of hamburgers or chicken nuggets. Vegetarian eating emphasizes whole foods prepared naturally, with minimum preservatives and low levels of added oils and sugars. So don't think that you're eating vegetarian style if all you're doing is sticking to the nonmeat side of the fast-food menu. You may feel virtuous by saying no to that burger, but what you're replacing it with aren't the best choices either.

The key to getting all the nutrients you need is eating a well-balanced vegetarian diet that emphasizes a wide variety of food selections. Problems can arise if you don't eat an assortment of plant proteins. For starters, you run the risk of not taking in enough calories. Plus, you might not get all the protein you need. If you're going to be a vegetarian athlete, you'll need to learn how to choose foods that will benefit your performance and promote your overall health.

Learning How to Eat Like a Vegetarian

Remember our old friend, the food pyramid? Well, there is a food pyramid for vegetarians that can help you learn how to make the best plant-based food choices. It works just like the other food pyramid. It's organized in similar fashion as well, with grains forming the base of the pyramid. Oils, fats, sweets, and salt—yes, salt!—are at the top of the pyramid and are to be eaten sparingly.

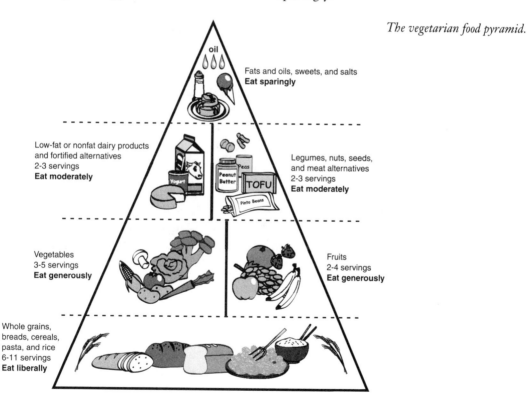

The vegetarian food pyramid.

What's most important is choosing foods that will help you meet your protein needs, as it's important that vegetarian athletes eat as much of this vital macronutrient as meat eaters do. For the most part, if you get good at this, you won't have to worry about taking in enough calories. Here are some ways to do it:

♦ Eat beans! Include legumes in salads. Use a variety of beans, including kidney beans, chickpeas, black beans, great northern beans, etc. They can have as much as 7 to 10 grams of protein per serving.

♦ Add texturized soy protein to pasta sauce, chili, or casseroles.

♦ Snack on healthy nuts, such as almonds, macadamias, and cashews. Yes, they're high in fat, so go easy on them, but research shows that they're good for you, too, as they contain cholesterol-lowering unsaturated fatty acids, antioxidant vitamins, minerals, and fibers.

♦ Make protein shakes with soft tofu or nondairy frozen desserts combined with fresh or frozen fruit and soy or rice milk.

♦ Add a quick protein boost to lunches and dinners with marinated tempeh or veggie burgers on a bun.

♦ Bake with soy flour or add powdered soy protein to baked goods. You'll have to experiment with the latter, however, as many soy powders can taste somewhat gritty or chalky.

> **Dawn Says**
>
> You don't have to give up your vegetarian diet when you're on the go. Many retailers stock vegetarian sports bars, soy shakes, and fruit shakes fortified with tofu or soy yogurt. Some even have vegan energy bars and other products.

The Veggie Shopping Cart

Vegetarian eating emphasizes whole foods prepared naturally, with minimum levels of added oils, salt, and sugars. When food shopping, you'll be filling your cart with things like the following:

♦ Dried beans and legumes

♦ Fresh fruit

♦ Fresh vegetables

♦ Whole-grain breads, as well as other whole grains such as bulgur wheat

♦ Whole-wheat pasta

♦ Soy-based dairy products, such as soy milk, soy yogurt, and soy cheese.

♦ Soy-based meat substitutes such as soy burgers, soy hot dogs, soy sausages, etc.

◆ Tofu or soy cakes

◆ Vegetarian convenience foods, such as frozen entrées, cups of soup, etc.

◆ Nuts and seeds, as well as products made from them such as peanut butter and tahini

If you're following a lacto-ovo vegetarian eating plan, you'll also buy eggs and dairy products.

> ### Dawn Says
> Vegetarian eating used to mean doing it yourself all the way, but there are more pre-pared and prepackaged vegetarian products hitting the market all the time. Even the smallest and most remote grocery store is bound to have some frozen vegetarian entrées and some soup cups. Some can be pretty tasty, while others not so. If you hit a "blecch" in your selections, don't give up on these products. Try other brands to see if they better suit your taste buds.

All About Soy

As you can tell by the previous list of foods, soy products play a big role in vegetarian eating. They are a great source of plant protein as well as calcium and iron. Including them in your meals will go a long way to ensuring that you're getting adequate levels of all of them.

Soy is also one of the more versatile food products out there. It can be made into veggie burgers, cheese, frozen desserts, sausages, and milk, just for starters. If you buy unflavored soy products, they'll take on the same flavor as the foods you put them with. Products to choose from include the following:

◆ Tofu. This is the soy product that most people are familiar with, as it's a staple in Chinese and Japanese cooking. You'll also see it in some Indian dishes. It's made from the curds that are left over from soy milk production and can be used a variety of ways. There are three types of tofu:

1. Firm tofu is thick and dense, which makes it great for stir-fry dishes and marinating. It also crumbles well. There is also extra-firm tofu, but you can make it yourself by putting firm tofu in a colander and placing a heavy object on top of it (protect the tofu with a plate or a paper towel or two first).

2. Soft tofu is less dense and is often used in soups or as a substitute for cheese in Italian dishes like manicotti and lasagna.

3. Silken tofu is extremely soft, almost creamy in texture, and works great in smoothies, dips, and other soft dishes. Silken tofu is also lower in fat than the other kinds.

◆ Soy milk. Soy milk comes plain or flavored. There are a number of different varieties and they don't all taste the same, so you might have to try a few to see what you like. If you don't care for any of them very much, you can still use soy milk. Just don't drink it straight—add it to smoothies or pour it over cereal. There is also low-fat soy milk.

◆ Soy yogurt. Made from soy milk, soy yogurt comes in a variety of flavors. Plain soy yogurt can be substituted for sour cream.

◆ Textured soy protein (TSP). Also called textured vegetable protein (TVP). This meat-substitute product is made from defatted soy flour. You'll find it in granules, chunks, and flakes, either plain or flavored. Use it like you would meat in things like tacos, chili, vegetarian casseroles, stews, and veggie burgers.

◆ Isolated soy protein. This is soy in powder form and it's the most protein packed of all the soy products—92 percent pure protein, in fact—as most of the fat and carbohydrate has been removed. It blends well into baked products—pancakes, muffins, cookies, and is a great way to sneak some plant proteins into the foods your family eats.

◆ Soy frozen desserts. These nondairy desserts are made from soy milk or soy yogurt. They come in a variey of flavors.

◆ Soy flour. Soy flour is made from roasted soybeans that are ground into a fine powder. If you're looking for a highly concentrated protein source, choose defatted soy flour, which has the highest protein levels.

◆ Soybeans. Available dried, roasted, fresh, or frozen. The fresh and frozen beans often go by edamame, their Japanese name. Edamame is fun to eat right out of the pod; roasted soybeans, either plain or flavored, are a great crunchy snack. Soybeans can also be added (once they're shelled) to lots of different recipes and are a great addition to salads, vegetable dishes, and stir-fry.

◆ Tempeh. Tempeh is a fermented soybean product that some people find easier to digest than other soy-based foods. It has a smoky or nutty flavor and can be substituted for meat in many recipes.

- Miso. Miso is a rich, salty paste made from soybeans and a grain such as rice. It is salted, cultured, and then aged for one to three years. Miso soup is a staple of the Japanese diet and is often eaten for breakfast. Miso can also be used to flavor dressings, sauces, and marinades.

- Natto. Natto is cooked and fermented whole soybeans. Because it's fermented, many people find natto easier to digest than whole soybeans. However, natto is definitely an acquired taste for many Westerners, largely due to its consistency. In Asian countries, natto is often used in miso soups and as a topping for rice.

> **Dawn Says**
>
> An unfortunate side effect of eating vegetarian style is—okay, I have to say it—flatulence. It's caused by increased dietary fiber and oligosaccharides, the complex carbohydrates found in beans that make them hard to digest for some people. If you're sensitive to beans and fiber, you'll want to back off them before you exercise and especially before major competitions. The biggest culprits are legumes, whole-grain products, dried fruit, and bran products.

Cooking Vegetarian Style

If you haven't followed a vegetarian diet before, it can take some time to learn how to prepare vegetarian dishes. Buying a couple of vegetarian cookbooks can be extremely helpful if you're a complete rookie at it. There are also several magazines that support vegetarian lifestyles. You'll find them listed in Appendix B. For some vegetarian recipes to get you started, turn to Chapter 4.

The Least You Need to Know

- It's perfectly healthy for athletes to be vegetarians and there is even evidence that a vegetarian diet can be a better energy boost than one that emphasizes animal proteins.

- Be sure to eat a variety of plant-based foods to ensure adequate calorie and protein levels.

- Soy products are the protein stars for vegetarians. Adding them to a variety of foods is an easy way to boost protein consumption.

- Knowing which foods to eat will help maintain important levels of micronutrients like calcium, iron, zinc, and B12.

- It's not necessary to eat certain combinations of plant foods at the same time to get complete proteins. Just eat a wide variety of them during the course of a day.

Part 5

Nutrition for Special Needs

People who are active are usually in better shape—both body composition-wise and weight-wise—than those who are not. Still, some athletes fight the battle of the bulge just like less active people do. Others have the opposite problem. Try as they might, they just can't add muscle to their wiry frames.

In this part, we'll explore the right way to lose weight—or, better put, the right way to lose fat, not muscle—and how optimizing your eating and your workouts can "bulk you up." Finally, you'll learn how to put your sports-nutrition knowledge to work to get back on your feet after illness or injury.

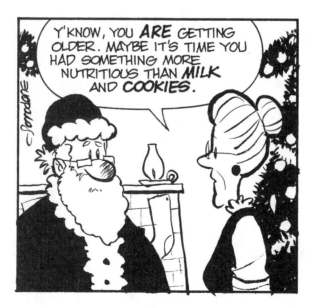

Chapter 22

Weight Loss and the Athlete

In This Chapter

◆ The formula for weight loss

◆ Learning how to factor calorie intake

◆ Losing weight the right way

◆ Best weight-loss tips

You'd have to be living under a rock, or just waking up from a nap of Rip Van Winklean proportions, to not know that obesity is becoming a serious problem in our world.

While people who are active tend to be in better shape both in body composition and weight than more sedentary people, losing weight or maintaining a proper weight is a concern for active people as well. The problem is, more and more people are failing at the battle of the bulge each year. As they do, they put themselves at increased risk of developing a battery of serious health problems, among them heart disease, diabetes, and cancer.

In this chapter we'll look at why obesity has become such an overwhelming concern. We'll also discuss the special dietary needs of overweight athletes and explore some ways to reduce fat and improve health and performance.

A Weighty Problem

Obesity has become a worldwide problem, with more than 300 million people considered to be obese and another 750 million overweight. Of all the countries in the world, however, the United States has taken the cake. America is a nation of plenty and our plenteousness extends to our waistlines. Over the past decade, obesity rates in all age groups have reached epidemic levels in the United States. Researchers have identified a number of reasons behind our surge in avoirdupoisity, but for the majority of people the weighty problem basically boils down two factors: they eat too much and they don't get enough exercise.

> **Dawn Says**
>
> When you're trying to lose weight, what you really want to focus on is losing fat. The key to success when it comes to decreasing the amount you weigh, and keeping it off, is losing fat, not muscle. So, whenever you see the term "weight loss," think "fat loss."

> **Eat It Up!**
>
> Research shows that losing weight through a combination of diet and exercise is more likely to lead to healthy blood lipid levels than simply cutting dietary fat alone.

Carrying too much weight in the form of excess body fat, of course, detracts from good health, physical fitness, and athletic performance. But it can also be deadly. An estimated 300,000 people every year die prematurely from a condition related to being overweight or obese.

Most athletes work extremely hard to keep their body-fat levels within the optimal ranges for their specific activities. If they're serious competitors, this is a must, because just an extra five pounds can make a difference between winning and losing. Many other people take up exercise as an adjunct to a weight-reduction diet, as a way to control their weight and improve their health. Some are successful at maintaining healthy levels of body fat. Some are not. Those who are not might be battling factors beyond their control when it comes to long-term weight maintenance. While you can't blame every little thing on genetics, researchers have proven that inherited genetic factors greatly influence body-fat distribution as well as the long-term programming of body size.

What we now know is that losing weight is a complicated process. It doesn't just come about through a combination of diet and exercise. It also depends on the right mix of nutrients, eating at the right times, eating enough, getting enough fiber—the list goes on. Some people have metabolisms that are so messed up that they have to get them back up first before they can even begin to decrease fat. When these factors are all taken into account, some people don't even need to decrease their calorie intake. They just need to make other changes that will help their bodies burn what they do take in more efficiently.

Reducing body fat should be the goal of virtually all weight-reduction plans. Losing both fat and muscle is only called for in situations when it's desirable to have a lighter body mass and a lower level of fat, such as when competing in weight-bearing endurance activities like running, racewalking, cross-country skiing, gymnastics, and ice skating. For these individuals, success in competition means honing their bodies into their ideal weight and composition. Carrying too much weight will slow them down. However, they can be thin but carry too much fat in proportion to their lean mass and this doesn't do them any good either.

Before we talk about ways to reduce fat while maintaining lean body mass, let's take a closer look at what body fat is all about.

> **Dawn Says**
>
> Decreasing calories is not always the right thing to do. I highly suggest that everyone see a dietitian who specializes in sports nutrition before embarking on a weight-loss program.

Chewing the Fat

Body fat is cellular tissue that primarily stores lipids. These fat-storing cells are contained in a web of connective tissue that separates them from muscle cells.

> **Dawn Says**
>
> While you might sometimes hear people say that their muscle turned to fat when they quit working out, this can't happen. Fat and muscle are two completely different kinds of tissue. Muscle is metabolically active, while fat is not. In other words, muscle is capable of burning energy, while fat can't. What does happen is that the muscle tissue shrinks in size because it's no longer being challenged to maintain its volume or to grow in size, and fat stores become more obvious. If eating fewer calories doesn't accompany lower activity levels and muscle loss, these fat stores also get larger as the calorie-burning muscle tissue shrinks. But this only happens during an extended period of time without activity—not in a day or a week.

Fat comes in two forms. Brown adipose tissue (BAT) is the tissue that regulates body temperature. It is prominent in mammals that hibernate; since humans don't hibernate, we don't have much of it. Instead, we have white adipose tissue.

Fat plays many roles in the body. It …

- ◆ Cushions the internal organs.
- ◆ Insulates the body.
- ◆ Stores fuel.
- ◆ Produces estrogen and helps regulate other hormones.

The fat in your body consists of essential fat and storage fat. Essential fat is the fat that's present in your organs, bone marrow, and nerve tissue. Instead of storing energy, essential fat assists essential bodily functions, hence the name. Storage fat is the fat that lies under your skin, and, in some people, around their organs. This is your energy reserve.

Dawn Says
The average man has about 3 percent essential fat and 12 percent storage fat, for a total of 15 percent body fat. The average woman has 12 percent essential fat—the higher number is related to childbearing and hormonal functions—and 15 percent storage fat, for a total of 27 percent body fat. It is impossible to stay healthy if body fat drops below the essential fat level.

We all have a certain amount of fat cells in our bodies that, to a certain extent, is determined by our genetic programming. These cells look somewhat like small balloons. And, just like balloons, they can be inflated or deflated.

The actual number of fat cells that the body contains can vary quite a bit from person to person. This number will remain fairly constant throughout adulthood if we stay within a reasonable range of weight for our height and build. But fat cells can and do multiply if you take in more calories than your body can use and you do so for an extended period of time. What's worse, once these fat cells multiply, they don't go away unless they're physically removed.

When you lose weight by decreasing the amount of fat that is stored in your fat cells, the cells don't miraculously disappear. They just lose their lipid volume and they deflate. Because they never go away, they can be reinflated. Once you gain these extra fat cells, it will always be easier for you to gain weight.

Losing Body Fat

For a long time, experts believed that people could lose excess weight simply by taking in fewer calories than they expended. But research has shown that the calories in/calories out equation is just part of the picture. We now know that genetics play a role in weight loss, and that it takes more than just eating less to lose weight. There are also techniques besides simply restricting calories and increasing exercise than can enhance weight loss and ensure that the pounds that drop are composed of the right stuff.

The goal in an effective weight-loss program is to lose no more than two pounds a week. Losing more than this indicates that muscle—the metabolically active tissue—is also being lost.

Dawn Says
If you are losing more than two pounds a week on a weight-loss program, you'll need to increase your calorie intake to reduce your rate of loss. Some people, however, can do everything right and still have a difficult time decreasing body fat. For these reasons, everyone who is embarking on a weight-loss plan should consult with his or her physician first and have the following levels checked: glucose, blood, homocyteine, and thyroid. Many of my clients who have thyroid problems, but now are normal because of medicine, still have a difficult time decreasing body fat in significant amounts.

Setting a Realistic Goal

Before you start on a weight-loss plan, it's a good idea to set a realistic goal for how much you want to lose. The simplest way to do this is to compare what you weigh to a chart that states the ideal weights for various heights and frames (small, medium, and large). However, this is about the worst approach you could take. Height and weight charts only reflect total body mass, and they're based on data drawn from an average population. They can't and don't take into account how much of total body mass is fat and how much is lean tissue. Two people who both weigh 150 can, and often do, have very different levels of body fat. One might be overweight, the other might not.

Athletes, in particular, often carry more muscle and have denser bones. They might technically be overweight if all they went by was the numbers they saw on the scale. Since the goal in weight loss is to lose body fat while retaining lean body mass, a far better way of determining how much weight you need to lose is to assess your ratio of fat to lean tissue.

There are several ways to determine this ratio. The following are the most common:

◆ Factoring *body mass index*. Body mass index, which uses weight and height to estimate the percentage of body fat in the body, has received a great deal of attention in the past few years and it's all but replaced the older weight and height charts as a standard measurement of general fitness and wellness. For athletic people, however, BMI doesn't cut it, because it doesn't take into account lean body mass or body frame. Someone who has a large frame and carries more muscle than the average individual could have a high BMI number and still be fit and lean.

Foodie

Body mass index, or **BMI,** is a formula that uses weight and height to estimate body fat and gauge health risks that can occur when carrying too much weight.

BMI can be determined by looking it up on a table or using a calculator. There are also a number of online BMI calculators. If you want to do it by hand, divide your weight in pounds by your height in inches. Then, divide this number by your height in inches again and multiply by 703. For example: If you weigh 130 and you are 5 feet 5 inches tall, your BMI would be 21.6. Based on the following chart, this weight would be well within desirable range.

Underweight	BMI less than 19
Desirable	BMI between 19 and 25
Increased health risks	BMI between 26 to 29
Obese	BMI between 30 and 40
Extremely obese	BMI over 40

◆ Bioelectrical impedance. Bioelectrical impedance measures the amount of water you have in your body with a tiny electrical current—50 KHz—as it moves through the body (it's painless). If you have a body-fat scale, this is exactly what goes on when you weigh yourself. Since muscle contains water, and water conducts electricity, the current moves faster through muscle than it does fat. This measurement can also be a less-than-accurate indication of body fat since your hydration level can affect readings. The margin of error can be as much as plus or minus 5 percent, which can mean a little or a lot, depending on the individual needing the information.

◆ Hydrostatic weighing. Hydrostatic weighing, or underwater weighing, determines body density and estimates the percentage of body fat based on the different densities of fat and fat-free tissues in the body. If you have this done, you'll first be weighed on dry land. Then you'll sit on a special seat in a tank of water and expel all the air from your lungs. As you do, you're lowered into the water until all your body parts are submerged. Then you're weighed again. Hydrostatic weighing, if done correctly, is the most accurate. The problem is finding a facility that's set up to do it. The equipment is expensive, and it's usually only found at research centers and hospitals.

◆ "Pinch-an-Inch." Skin-fold measurements done with calipers are another common gauge of body fat. The skin is pinched at various spots on the body, usually at the triceps, the waist, and the thigh. The information is then plugged into a calculator for analysis. This test can be fairly accurate if it's done by someone who knows what he or she is doing. However, the margin of error with this test is still fairly high.

Some people determine how much they should weigh by taking their measurements—bust or chest, waist, and hips—and basing their weight-loss efforts on how much they deviate from what they think is ideal. Bad idea! Not only are tape measurements extremely inaccurate, basing your weight-loss program on how your measurements stack up is simply unrealistic. Very few people have ideal measurements. If you tend to be a bit of a pear shape, for example, you could be at your ideal weight and still be comparatively large below the waist.

What all of these methods will give you is an indication of how much fat you're carrying around. This figure will be expressed as a percentage of body weight; i.e., if you weigh 180 and you've been told that your level of body fat is 30 percent, this would mean that of your 180 pounds, 54 of them are fat. The remainder—126 pounds—is your lean body mass, or LBM. This is the number you want to maintain when you lose weight.

As an example, let's say that you're the person we've just described, and you want to reduce your percentage of body fat to 25, which would be at the high end of the range. So you go on a diet and you manage to lose 30 pounds, which puts you at 150. You're feeling pretty good at this point, so you go in to have your body fat measured. You find out that you hit your mark—you're now down to 25 percent body fat. Of the 150 pounds you're now carrying around, 37.5 of them are fat and 112.5 are LBM. What you now know is that you lost some lean body tissue along with that fat—just under 14 pounds of it—but you also lost 12.5 pounds of fat. That's not bad, but it could be better.

Another possible scenario has you losing the same amount of weight, but you overshot your goal when it came to decreasing body fat and you find out that it's down to 20 percent. You only lost 30 pounds of fat, compared to 37.5 in the first example, but you kept your LBM pretty close to where it was before. This is a far better outcome. Not only have you decreased your percentage of body fat, but you've also maintained a good level of LBM, and it's this lean body mass that will help you keep the weight off.

If you're an athlete who competes in a sport where weight is an issue, have a sports nutritionist or a trainer do a body-fat assessment to determine what your ideal level would be for your sport. Different sports have different requirements. For example, contact sports and sports that require muscle power usually necessitate large body mass and low body fat. Weight-bearing endurance sports like marathons require a lighter body mass and a lower level of body fat. If you just like to be fit and active, you should do well if you stay on the low end of the averages for men and women.

The normal and ideal ranges for body fat are different for men and women, with the percentages for women being higher than those for men. As previously stated, the average man has 15 percent body fat and the average woman has 27 percent body fat. For general good health, men should aim for between 10 to 15 percent body fat. For women, 20 to 25 percent is considered ideal.

Foodie

The energy contained in food is measured in terms of **calories**. Technically, one calorie is the amount of energy it takes to increase the temperature of 1 gram of water by 1 degree Centigrade. The calorie measure that's used to describe the energy content of food is actually a kilocalorie, or 1,000 calories, which is the amount of energy required to raise one kilogram of water (about 2.2 pounds) by one degree Centigrade.

These figures, however, are for average individuals, not for athletes. Many competitive athletes go lower than this. Competitive bodybuilders drop their body fat to amazingly low levels before competition—around 5 percent in men and below 10 percent in women. However, it's almost impossible for them to stay at such low levels, because their bodies won't let them do it for long. Their metabolisms will slow and their hormone levels will switch over to starvation mode to preserve what little body fat they have left.

Factoring Calories

The next step in putting together an effective weight-loss program is figuring out how many *calories* you need to eat to put your body into calorie-deficit mode.

Since it takes 3,500 calories to make up a pound of fat, the simplest approach is to decrease the amount of calories you eat a day by 500. This alone should help you lose one pound a week. Any other weight that comes off would be the result of increasing your activity level beyond where it currently is. Keep in mind, though, that successful fat loss also depends on other factors such as when you eat and the kinds of food that you eat. Figuring out how many calories you should eat is a good starting point, however.

Dawn Says

Whenever I work with a client who wants to lose weight, I always have him or her keep a seven-day food record so that I can compare the calories they actually eat on a daily basis to what they think they're taking in. I also use the food record to track the types of food he or she eats, the percentages of carbs, proteins, and fats; the amount of vitamins and minerals; fluid intake; fiber intake; when they eat; how much they eat; and how they mix their meals.

To do this computation, you'll have to determine how many calories you eat daily. The easiest way to do this is to keep a food journal in which you write down everything you eat, how much you eat, and how many calories these foods contain.

A more complex approach to knowing how much you need to eat requires determining the following factors:

◆ Your basal metabolic rate, or BMR, which is the amount of energy your body needs to fuel itself while at complete rest.

◆ Your activity level.

◆ The number of calories you need to digest food.

Tests that accurately measure BMR are generally pretty expensive. However, you can get an idea of what your BMR is by following this formula:

1. Multiply your body weight by 10 if you're a woman, and by 11 if you're a man. For example, if you weigh 150, this first figure would be 1,500 for a woman and 1,650 for a man.

2. Calculating your activity level. If you're inactive, you'd multiply your BMR calories from step 1 by 30 percent; if moderately active, multiply by 50 percent; if very active, multiply by 75 percent.

3. Next, calculate the calories you need to digest food by adding your BMR calories to your activity calories and multiplying by 0.1.

4. Finally, add the results from each step.

As an example, let's say you're a woman who weighs 155. Your first figure would be 1,550. You think you're fairly active, so you multiply this figure by 75 percent to get 1,162.5. Next, you calculate the calories you need to digest food by adding 1,550 (your BMR calories) to 1,162.5 (your activity calories) and multiplying by 0.1 to get 271.25. Finally, you add all the numbers together: 1,550+1,162.5+271.25=2,983.75.

This final number—2,983.75—is the amount of calories you would need to eat to maintain your weight. To lose weight, you'd eat below it. To gain weight, you'd eat above it. In general, you never want to eat less than 500 to 1,000 calories below your BMR or 500 to 1,000 calories above your BMR.

This is the most common way to calculate calorie needs, and it does a pretty good job. Here's another way to factor your intake level that's even more accurate:

1. Calculate your resting metabolism by multiplying your weight by 11 if you're a woman, or by 12 if you're a man. This is the amount of calories you burn when you're at complete rest.

2. Next, multiply this number by your activity level:

   Sedentary (no formal exercise and a sit-down job): BMR x .25

   Active (three hours of aerobic activity a week, no sit-down job): BMR x .50

   Very Active (an athlete who exercises several hours a day): BMR x .75.

3. The next calculation takes into account what you eat.

   For a high-fat diet (40 percent of calories from fat): BMR x .05

   For a high-carb diet (60 percent of calories from carbohydrates): BMR x .1.

4. Calculate total energy expenditure by adding the figures you arrived at in steps 1, 2, and 3.

5. The final calculation is what sets this method of factoring calorie intake apart from the other. What you want to do is adjust the figure you arrived at in step 4 to take into account the amount of lean tissue in your body. Here's why: If you carry more fat than the average person, you need to take in fewer calories. If you are lower in body fat than normal, you burn more energy and can eat more.

This last calculation gets a little tricky, but here's how it's done. First, you'll need to know your body composition—your percentages of fat and lean tissue. Next, you'll subtract the average for your sex from this figure. For example, if you are a woman at 30 percent body fat, you'd subtract 22 percent (the female average for body fat) from 30 percent for a total of 8 percent. If you're a man, base this calculation on the male average of 18 percent body fat.

Next, subtract the difference between actual body fat and average body fat from 100. Multiply the figure you reached in step 4 by this number.

As an example, let's do this calculation for a man who weighs 185, has 20 percent body fat, is moderately active, and eats a diet that's high in carbohydrates:

Resting metabolism: $185 \times 12 = 2{,}220$

Energy burn: $185 \times .50 = 92.5$

Dietary factor: $185 \times .10 = 18.5$

Total energy expenditure: $2{,}220 + 92.5 + 18.5 = 2{,}331$

Lean tissue adjustment: $100\% — (20\% – 18\%) = 98\%$

$2{,}331 \times .98 = 2{,}284$

2,284 is the amount of calories this man needs to maintain his weight.

Building Your Weight-Loss Program

Now that you know how much you want to lose, and how many calories you need to eat in a day to facilitate that loss, you can customize a weight-loss program to meet your needs. Here's how to do it:

1. First, start by determining how many grams of protein you need to eat every day. This figure should be based on the amount of body fat you want to lose and what your lean muscle mass currently is. Protein needs can vary greatly depending on individual goals, especially if you are trying to gain muscle at the same time you're losing fat. To come up with the best figure for protein consumption, it's a good idea to meet with a nutritionist or dietitian who can fine-tune the numbers to meet your specific needs.

2. Next, add some carbohydrates to that protein. Choose from all the carbohydrate categories. If you need help, refer back to the food pyramid in Chapter 6. You want a 45-60:20-30 balance of carbs to protein. The remaining 20 percent of your calorie intake per day will come from fat. You'll get most of what you need from the protein you eat, plus maybe a little additional fat that you'll use in preparing your meals. Be sure to include at least three to four servings of vegetables and two to three fruits every day. Again, the exact balance of protein to carbohydrates varies depending on individual needs. Some people do well with carbs at around 50 percent, protein at 20 to 25 percent, and healthy fat at 20 to 30 percent. Remember, fat and protein make you feel full and also help to release energy slowly into the bloodstream. Again, meeting with a dietitian or nutritionist will help you determine the levels that are right for your needs.

Dawn Says

When choosing carbohydrates, pick ones that will give you between 20 to 40 grams of fiber a day. Fiber not only helps clean out your pipes, it also takes longer to absorb, so you'll feel fuller longer. Also, make sure you pick a good mix of carbohydrates. Many people fall into the trap of eating what I call "easy carbs," things like bagels, rice cakes, and pretzels that are low in fiber and high on the glycemic index. This is the worst thing you can do when you're trying to lose weight. You'll get hungry faster, you won't feel as full, and you'll be missing out on important nutrients from the other food groups.

3. Now, put together a menu that includes eating at least four times a day—breakfast, lunch, and dinner, plus a snack. If you want to keep your body fueled even better, plan for three meals and two snacks. If you're working out regularly (and you should be), you might plan to eat one of your snacks before you work out. Eating frequently will help you burn more energy, and, in turn, more fat. The goal is to be eating every three to four hours.

If you need some help with healthy food choices and menu planning, go to Chapters 3 and 16.

Making the Best Food Choices

When you're following a reduced-calorie eating program, you want to make sure that every calorie you do eat is the best you can be putting into your mouth. This means selecting foods that are high in nutritional value and low in fat. Your best choices will include:

◆ Low-fat animal protein such as chicken or turkey breasts, pork, and beef.

◆ Seafood and shellfish.

◆ Low-fat dairy products such as cottage cheese, milk, and yogurt. Many cheese products, even those that are low in fat, are high in sodium, so try to minimize these in your eating program.

◆ Vegetables with dark, rich colors. The darker the veggie, the better the nutrient value. Aim for a wide variety of vegetables in your eating program. If you're not much of a vegetable fan, stick to the ones you know you like. Try something new each week.

◆ Fruit instead of fruit juice. The fiber in fruit helps it stay in your system longer and prevents blood sugar spikes.

◆ Whole grains and products made from whole grains, such as whole-wheat pasta, crackers, breads, and the like. Make sure your selections are low in fat as well.

◆ Beans and legumes. Both are great sources of plant protein as well as being low in fat and high in fiber.

Any oils or spreads you add to your eating plan should be as high in unsaturated fat as possible. Also choose products with no trans-fatty acids.

Using the Glycemic Index

As mentioned in Chapter 7, carbohydrates range in how quickly they'll trigger a spike in blood sugar. Foods that have a high GI break down quickly during digestion and cause a fast response; those that are low on the GI index break down more slowly and release glucose more gradually into your system. Knowing the glycemic index of the foods you eat, and choosing foods that have low glycemic indexes, will help you lose weight faster. Here's why: When you eat them, your blood sugar will stay more stable and you won't get hungry as often.

In general, foods in their whole state—whole grains, whole fruits, and whole vegetables—are lower in glycemic index than foods that are processed.

Watering It All Down

Staying hydrated is always essential for maintaining good health. When you're trying to lose weight, those eight to ten glasses of water you're drinking will also help you control your appetite. If you find you're still hungry after eating a meal, chase that meal with a large glass of water. Chances are good that it will slake any lingering hunger pangs you might have.

Water also plays a key role in moving nutrients, vitamins, and minerals around in your body and in removing waste products from it. If you don't drink enough water, you'll slow down cell function, which in turn slows down weight loss. Just increasing water intake can jump-start a weight-loss program that has hit a plateau.

Monitoring Portion Sizes

Being aware of how much food you eat by monitoring your portion sizes is important both while you're losing weight and when you're maintaining your loss. It isn't necessary to measure out everything you eat, but you do need to learn how to eyeball things so you can tell whether you're eating too much, not enough, or just right. As a refresher, a portion of most foods—salad, pasta, rice, meat, chicken, etc.—should be no larger than your clenched fist.

Working Off the Calories

Exercise is another component of a successful weight-loss program. Without it, you'll lose muscle along with fat, which is exactly what you don't want to do. Remember, it's muscle, not fat, that burns calories. The more muscle you have, the more you can eat and the less you'll have to worry about gaining weight.

Both aerobic exercise and resistance training are important for weight loss. Aerobic activities such as running, walking, bicycling, exercise classes, and so on burn calories faster than resistance training, and they're essential for maintaining good cardiovascular health. However, it's better to emphasize resistance training when you're trying to lose weight. It doesn't burn as many calories as aerobic activities do. However, aerobics don't build muscle. Resistance training does.

> **Dawn Says**
>
> The average person loses between $1/2$ to 1 pound of muscle a year, starting at age 30. By adding muscle and preventing muscle loss, you'll burn more calories every day.

The goal is to expend at least 1,000 calories a week doing cardiovascular activities that get your heart rate up to between 50 to 85 percent of your maximum rate. These workouts should be done 4 to 6 times a week for 30 to 60 minutes. If you're working out at a lower intensity, do longer sessions. If you're at higher intensities, go shorter.

For suggestions on putting together a resistance-training program, turn to Chapter 23.

When you exercise and what you eat before and after you exercise can influence the amount of fat your body uses for energy during exercise. Training in the morning before you eat anything increases the amount of fat you burn. However, this amount will also depend on the kind of shape you're in. If you're not well trained to begin with, your muscles won't be as efficient at using fat for energy as they would be if you were in condition. Doing so also comes with some risks. You could develop hypoglycemia due to low blood sugar and you put yourself at greater risk for getting sick as you could compromise your immune system.

The best approach seems to be eating a light, high-carb snack before your workout, or drinking a sports drink before and after.

The Least You Need to Know

- More people are failing at the battle of the bulge each year and are at increased risk of developing heart disease, diabetes, and cancer.

- The calories in/calories out equation is just part of weight loss.

- Losing up to two pounds a week is a realistic goal. A faster rate of loss than this means that muscle is being lost along with fat.

- Combining aerobic exercise, resistance training, and a calorie-reduced eating program is the best way to lose weight while retaining as much lean body mass as possible.

Chapter 23

Fat to Muscle

In This Chapter

- The components of a weight-gaining program
- Avoiding fat gain
- Protein needs for building muscle
- Eating strategies for muscle gain
- Lifting weights for muscle gain

While many athletes are concerned about decreasing body fat, others have exactly the opposite problem and need to add some mass to their frames.

To everyone who has done battle with the scale in trying to get his or her numbers to go down instead of up, having to gain muscle mass seems like it would be a cakewalk. Just eat more calories and the weight will pop right on. This is true to a certain extent if you don't care what kind of weight you gain. However, to gain weight right, you want to build muscle, not lay on fat. And that means more than just opening your mouth and shoveling in the calories.

Weight Gain Challenges

Putting on muscle is simply easier for some people than it is for others. Many factors come into play, including:

- ◆ Age. Younger people have more of the hormones needed for putting on muscle than older folks do.

- ◆ Caloric intake. You have to eat more calories to put on weight, period.

- ◆ Stress. High levels of stress promote muscle breakdown, plus a lot more free radicals.

- ◆ Body type. Some people are just naturally built to be able to put on weight more easily than others.

- ◆ Sex. Not the act, the gender. Thanks to their higher levels of male hormones, men usually ace out women in their ability to pack on muscle mass.

- ◆ Muscle memory. If you've done any strength training at all, your muscles have something called muscle memory. They will remember what you've done and make it a little easier for you to restore your muscularity.

The challenge for anyone who is trying to gain weight is to put on the right kind of weight. The goal is to gain muscle weight, not fat weight. The training program you follow will also have a big impact on your ability to pack on muscle. We'll get into this later in this chapter.

A muscle-gaining program has three basic components. It involves the following:

- ◆ Increasing your calories

- ◆ Doing heavy resistance training with free weights

- ◆ Getting enough rest

The benefits of gaining muscle are many. Maintaining good muscle mass speeds up your metabolism and increases the level of good HDL cholesterol in your body. More muscle also increases your aerobic capacity as an additional muscle uses more oxygen. Exchanging fat for muscle can also help prevent type II diabetes, because that additional muscle will also take up extra sugar. Strength training also helps increase bone density and can help prevent osteoporosis.

Upping Your Calories

When you want to increase your size, you have to take in more calories than you burn. The ideal is to eat just enough calories to help your body build more muscle, but not so many calories that you end up storing them as large amounts of body fat. For some people, increasing their calorie intake to an extra 500 calories a day and taking in the right balance of protein, carbohydrates, and fats will do the trick. People who have trouble gaining size may have to boost their intake by as much as an additional 1,500 calories a day.

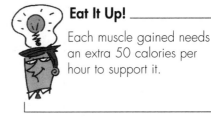

Eat It Up! _____

Each muscle gained needs an extra 50 calories per hour to support it.

Pumping Up the Protein

While most people, regardless of their activity level, are rarely lacking in protein, individuals who are working hard to build muscle have roughly twice the protein needs of the average person and generally need to add protein to their eating plans.

There are a number of good protein sources to choose from to boost your intake levels. What you want, however, are foods that are low in fat and are protein dense, such as the following:

♦ Whey protein. As discussed in Chapter 14, whey protein is the gold standard when it comes to protein supplements. It is rich in three of the essential amino acids—isoleucine, leucine, and valine—that comprise muscle protein, it is low in fat, and it enters the blood stream rapidly. It also has the highest biological value—meaning that more of it is absorbed—than other protein sources.

♦ Casein protein. Another important protein source for building muscle, casein protein works more slowly than whey protein does. Recent research suggests that using whey protein before training and casein protein after training speeds protein into the muscles for protein synthesis during the workout and minimizes protein breakdown after it.

> **Dawn Says**
>
> To gain muscle weight, you have to eat! Just as some people work hard to decrease body fat, you have to put as much effort into gaining muscle mass.

♦ Eggs. If you're worried about cholesterol, ditch the yolks and eat the whites. They have plenty of protein, no cholesterol, and no fat.

CAUTION

Food Foul-Ups

Unless you buy your eggs from a supplier you know and trust, never do the "Rocky" thing and eat eggs raw or undercooked. Doing so puts you at risk for salmonella poisoning. To kill salmonella, eggs must be boiled for at least seven minutes, poached for at least five minutes, or fried for at least three minutes per side. Scrambled eggs and omelets should be served dry, not runny.

♦ Chicken and turkey breasts. The white meat of chicken and turkey is a good source of low-fat protein if you eat it without the skin. Some people find chicken easier to digest than red meat. You can also buy ground chicken and turkey, but be careful when you do. Look for products that say "ground breast meat." Other ground poultry products can contain dark meat, skin, and organ meat.

♦ Lentils. One of the top plant-based proteins. One-half cup of lentils contains almost 9 grams of protein and almost 20 grams of carbohydrates. They're also a good source of fiber.

♦ Lean beef. Choose cuts that are lower in fat, like top round, eye of round, top sirloin, London broil, flank steak, and extra-lean ground beef or ground chuck. Trim all visible fat. Red meat is also a good source of heme iron and zinc. If you're looking for a break from beef, try buffalo or venison, which are even lower in fat than low-fat beef cuts are.

♦ Fish. Plain fish—that is, fish that isn't breaded or prepared with butter—is an excellent source of low-fat protein. Try salmon, tuna, haddock, cod, perch, halibut, snapper, swordfish, and sea bass. Shellfish such as crab, lobster, and scallops are also high in protein and low in fat. Although it's not a good idea to eat too much canned tuna fish due to the mercury content in tuna, one can of water-packed tuna has about 1 gram of fat and about 24 grams of protein.

♦ Protein bars. High-quality protein bars can pack as much as 25 to 50 grams of protein with little or no carbs or fat. They are a great way to boost your protein intake when time is short and you need to eat.

♦ Low-fat cottage cheese. Cottage cheese is the bodybuilder's favorite. It's rich in amino acids, including glutamine, which helps support muscle metabolism. What's more, no cooking is required. Just scoop and eat.

As a rule, in order to gain muscle mass, you need to eat at least 1.7 to 2.0 grams of protein per kg (2.2 lbs) of body weight for men, and 1.4 to 1.7 grams for women.

As an example, if you're a man weighing 175 pounds, you would need to eat somewhere in the range of 175 grams of protein. Keep in mind, though, that these recommendations are based on averages, and that there are many different ways to compute protein needs. If you're after the best results, you'll want to consult a dietitian or sports nutritionist at least once to make sure that what you're doing is the best you can do for yourself.

Depending on how much you weigh, the amount of protein you need can constitute as much as 18 to 30 percent of your total calorie intake for a day. No matter how you look at it, this is a heck of a lot of protein, especially when a normal level of protein intake is in the 70 to 80 gram range. The good news is that you won't be eating all that extra protein in one sitting.

> **CAUTION**
>
> **Food Foul-Ups**
>
> Consuming too much protein—more than 30 percent of your total daily calorie intake—can do more harm than good. Researchers have found that eating too much protein can stress the other systems in your body. Your kidneys, for example, have to work harder to flush the ketone buildup from your system that results from diets that sacrifice carbohydrates for protein.

Getting It All In

Packing on muscle also means having to eat more often. If you're already eating three meals and two snacks a day, you'll have to add another small meal or snack to your eating plan during your muscle-building phase. Some people up their snack/meal count to seven. If you're awake for 16 hours, this means you'll be eating something every two to three hours or so. Some people even make sure that their bodies stay fueled while they're asleep and get up in the middle of the night to eat.

It can be difficult to fit in six to seven meals a day, which is why many people who are on weight-gaining programs use protein supplements. Protein powders and bars are both good choices. There are tons of them out there and you may have to experiment a bit to find the ones that work for you and that you like the taste of.

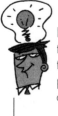

> **Eat It Up!**
>
> If you're going to use protein powders or bars purely as protein sources, look for those that are high in protein and have little or no carbs or fat. If you're using them as replacement meals, choose products that are high in carbohydrate and protein and low in fat. Ratios should be similar to real food—50 to 70 percent carbohydrate, 15 to 30 percent protein, and 5 to 30 percent fat.

Getting in all those extra calories also calls for planning ahead and for knowing how much you're actually eating. To be successful at gaining muscle, you must know how much protein, fat, and carbs you're eating each day. This is essential for helping you control exactly what goes into your body. Guessing does not work.

> ### Dawn Says
>
> I always recommend that my muscle-gaining clients measure their food out for a week. Doing this gives them a good idea of the portion sizes they need to eat for each meal. People who are trying to gain weight usually over-report what they eat, as opposed to people who are trying to lose weight, who usually under-report what they are eating. Use a food scale to accurately weigh your food quantities to help you monitor and control how much you eat.

Pre- and Post-Workout Eating Plans

Eating six to seven times a day means that you'll be eating a meal or snack pretty close to both sides of your workouts. What you eat at these times is important for fueling your muscle growth.

Before your workout …

Eat a whole-food meal or meal-replacement shake 60–120 minutes before training. This meal's carbohydrate (complex carb)-to-protein ratio should be approximately 1:1. The calorie count should be between 250 to 350 calories.

If you're eating a whole-food meal, try $1/2$ cup oatmeal and 4 ounces nonfat cottage cheese. The pregame meals in Chapter 16 also have the right mix of nutrients for pregame or practice meals. If you're using a meal replacement drink, choose one that falls in the same 1:1 carbohydrate-to-protein ratio.

After your workout …

Taking in the right balance of carbohydrates to protein is also important after you work out. Research has shown that carbohydrate and protein eaten within 30 minutes of a workout will help restore amino acids and carbohydrate to the muscles and help them prepare for the next workout.

Your post-workout meal should consist of about 50 grams of simple carbohydrates and 20 grams of protein. Here, a whey protein powder is a good choice as it is about as pure a protein source as you can get and your body absorbs it very quickly. Fruit is a great source of simple carbohydrates and is a good choice for this meal. The carbohydrate-to-protein ratio should be approximately 2:1. This is also the best time to take supplemental glutamine. The amount of carbohydrate and protein grams will vary depending on individual needs. For best results, consult with a dietitian who specializes in sports nutrition to fine-tune these numbers.

Within 30 minutes of your workout, make a fruit salad from $1/2$ small cantaloupe, 1 small apple, and 1 banana. Add whey protein or a protein bar. Then, about an hour to one and a half hours later, eat a second post-workout meal that contains complex carbohydrates and protein, such as chicken and vegetables with rice or pasta. The same ratio—2:1—applies to this meal as well. Add some healthy fat—olives, avocados, flaxseeds or oil, nuts, or seeds.

> **Dawn Says**
>
> Most people will gain some body fat as they gain muscle mass. This is especially so if you have a difficult time gaining muscle weight. When you get to your desired weight, or close to it, you can switch gears and work at decreasing the small amount of body fat you gained.

Weight Training

As previously mentioned, weight training or resistance training is essential for putting on weight and building muscle. It works synergistically with increasing calorie intake. Lifting weights challenges the muscles and stimulates growth, while the food you eat provides the necessary building blocks to repair and build new muscle tissue.

For the best results, resistance training should focus on lifting weights that are heavy enough to give your muscles a good challenge. Doing so will stimulate the greatest number of muscle fibers, which in turn increases muscle mass. Lifting free weights is the method of choice for fast muscle gain. Because there is no other structure or armature to support their weight besides your own body, you have to do the work throughout the entire movement. Not relying on a machine for assistance results in greater muscle stimulation. It also doesn't let smaller or weaker muscles off the hook as you'll have to use them all to lift and lower the weights correctly.

> **Eat It Up!**
>
> Lifting weights is the single best physical activity you can do for your body. As you grow older, you lose muscle mass—as much as six pounds per decade. As you lose muscle, your metabolism slows down and you can't eat as much as you did when you were younger. If you do, you'll gain weight. Maintaining good muscle mass means you can eat more calories without gaining fat.

Measuring Up

First and foremost, get a measuring tape. This is essential for keeping track of how much your body parts grow. Don't go by what you look like in those mirrors—your mind's eye can deceive you.

Fill in the chart below with your beginning measurements. Then take them every four to six weeks, and enter the changes.

Body Part	Starting Measurement
Waist	_____
Chest	_____
Left Bicep	_____
Right Bicep	_____
Left Forearm	_____
Right Forearm	_____
Left Thigh	_____
Right Thigh	_____
Left Calf	_____
Right Calf	_____

The reason for measuring both your left and right sides is to make sure that you're gaining symmetry as well as size. Most people will be a little larger on their dominant side as they use these muscles more. Don't worry if your measurements don't exactly match up—they usually won't. If there is a big difference between your sides, and it bothers you, you may want to schedule a few sessions with a personal trainer to see what you can do to even things out.

Dawn Says

People who have a difficult time gaining muscle mass usually need more rest and food than others. If you're having problems putting on muscle, keep track of how much you eat, how much you sleep, and how much you work out for about a week or so. Doing so might show you where your routine might need some tweaking. Be honest about what you record. Underreporting or overreporting only hurts you, not anyone else.

Working Out Right

You don't have to train like a maniac to get results. Lots of people think that more is better when it comes to weight lifting, and they'll spend hours in the weight room almost every day of the week in pursuit of massive biceps and ripped abs. (You have to wonder if they have lives outside of the gym, don't you?) But here's the truth about muscle growth: It happens after you work out, not in the gym. Weight training only stimulates muscle growth. After you're done lifting those weights, you need to give your muscles a chance to recover. Working out too often, and not allowing yourself adequate recovery times between workouts, doesn't give your muscles the time they need to recuperate and grow. In other words, you can actually lose muscle if you work out too often. And, you also set yourself up for chronic injuries from overtraining.

Gaining Mass, Strength, or Endurance

Everyone has different goals when it comes to weight training. Some people want bigger muscles; others want to increase their strength (the two don't necessarily go hand in hand). Others want to build endurance. The following table will give you an idea of what your strength-training routine should look like, based on your particular goals:

Goal	Resistance	Repetitions	Sets	Rest
Muscle Strength	Heavy	3–8	3–5	2–5 min.
Muscle Size	Moderate	8–12	3–5	30–90 sec.
Endurance	Light	12–20	2–3	15–30 sec.

If you want to gain mass, you'll need to use weights that are heavy enough that you have to stop at anywhere from six to ten repetitions, or reps. If you can do more, increase the weight the next time you work out.

If you are underweight, you probably have a very high metabolism, or you don't eat enough calories. To build muscle, you'll need to eat more calories, of course, but it's also a good idea to train less frequently but with more intensity, using the following table as a guideline:

Day	Exercise Type
Monday	Chest, Shoulders, Triceps
Tuesday	Rest
Wednesday	Back and Biceps
Thursday	Rest
Friday	Legs and Abs
Saturday	Rest
Sunday	Play sports or jog

This schedule works each muscle group once a week and allows plenty of time for the muscles to recover between workouts.

Getting Intense

Ask anyone who is serious about weight training, and has the body to prove it, how he or she got there, and chances are pretty good that you'll hear something along the lines of "You gotta work hard." What that means is that you have to put some effort into your workouts. In other words, you have to lift with intensity. In the weight-lifting world, this is called high-intensity training.

Intensity doesn't mean lifting weights so heavy that it feels like your head is going to explode when you heft them. Instead, when you lift with intensity, you maximize your workouts by making your muscles work hard in a short period of time with little recovery time during the workout. In other words, instead of lifting a 30 pound weight 30 times (10 reps × 3 sets), and resting for a few minutes between sets because you can't breathe, you'll instead lift a slightly lower weight—say, 25 pounds—the same amount of times but without taking as much time to recover. Or you can do more reps with the lighter weight in the same amount of time that you spent lifting the heavier weight less often. Here's how the exertion levels for each method compare:

30 lbs × 30 reps = 900 pounds lifted

900 lbs divided by 5 minutes (the amout of time it took you to lift) = 180 pounds per minute (this is your intensity level)

25 lbs × 30 reps = 750 pounds lifted

750 divided by 3 minutes (the amount of time it took you to lift) = 250 pounds per minute (intensity level)

25 lbs × 45 reps (three sets of 15 reps each) = 1,125 lbs lifted

1125 divided by 5 minutes (the amount of time it took you to lift) = 225 lbs per minute (intensity level)

If the concept of high-intensity training is new to you, you might want to consider scheduling a few sessions with a trainer so you can learn the proper techniques for doing it. It's not difficult, but it is important to know how to do this type of training correctly to get the best benefits from it and to avoid injuries.

Getting Enough Rest

After an intense resistance-training workout, your lean body mass will actually decrease. This happens because muscle-building is anaerobic, meaning that it doesn't use oxygen for fuel. Instead, it burns the contents of the muscles—glycogen, water, and minerals. In other words, your muscles actually break down when you stress them by lifting weights.

Gaining muscle requires giving your body enough time to synthesize muscle tissue to replace what it has burned up. New muscle must be synthesized at a higher rate than the old, burned-up stuff to result in an increase in muscle size.

The basic recommendation is to give each muscle group at least 24 hours' worth of rest before working it again. For better results, and especially when working out at high intensities, you'll want to give each group an even longer break—at least 48 hours. Many people who lift weights on a regular basis cycle their workouts so that they're working each body part only every three days or so.

Supplements for Weight Gain

There are two nutritional supplements that have been proven to enhance the body's ability to gain muscle. Creatine is currently one of the hottest ergogenic aids. Research shows that it increases strength and muscle endurance, which will let you lift more weight and, ultimately, build more muscle. While the average diet naturally contains some creatine, it usually doesn't have enough to support muscle growth. For this reason, supplementation is necessary. Most creatine manufacturers recommend taking a loading dose of 20 grams per day for 5 days, followed by a maintenance dose of 2 to 5 grams per day.

Glutamine is the other supplement that can help you pack on some muscle. Researchers have found that it not only helps maintain muscle mass, but it can also combat the muscle-wasting effects of stress hormones that are stimulated during intense exercise. The recommended dosage is 1 to 20 grams per day when you're doing high-intensity workouts.

> **Dawn Says**
>
> There is no scientific evidence to support the loading phase of creatine supplementation. Some research even suggests that a loading phase isn't necessary and that you'll get the same results if you just take the maintenance dose of 2 to 5 grams a day. Your weight gain might be slower, but a large weight gain over a short amount of time is usually water because it helps build muscle.

Keep in mind, though, that supplementation is never meant to replace a good eating plan and a solid weight-training program. Any supplements that you take should enhance your efforts in both areas, not replace them.

Like everything else when it comes to good health, building muscle takes time, effort, and discipline with what you eat and the workouts you do to enhance muscle gain. When you devote the time necessary to make both components of a muscle-building program the best that they can be, you'll see results. Supplements may simply help you reach your goals faster.

The Least You Need to Know

- ◆ Some people build muscle more easily than others.

- ◆ It takes approximately 1 gram of protein per pound of body weight to gain muscle mass.

- ◆ Gaining muscle requires eating more calories than you expend. This means eating a balanced diet that provides at least 300 to 500 calories more than what you need to maintain your weight.

- ◆ Weight training is the fastest way to put on muscle and one of the best things you can do to stay in shape, keep fit, and reduce stress.

- ◆ Eating the right foods at the right time can enhance your body's ability to build more muscle.

24

Getting Back on Your Feet

In This Chapter

- ◆ How the body responds to injury and illness
- ◆ The parts of the immune system
- ◆ The role of nutrition in recovery
- ◆ How antioxidants can help you heal faster

It can happen before you know it. You take a misstep during a workout, or you start to feel kind of under the weather after a race, and the next thing you know, you're off your feet with an injury, or you're sick in bed.

Unfortunately, the more active you are, and the more you compete in athletic events, the greater the chances of your getting injured somewhere along the line. And although athletes tend to be healthier than their more sedentary counterparts, they aren't immune to getting sick either. There are even certain times when they might be more susceptible to illness than their couch-sitting buddies are.

Getting sick or sustaining an injury happens to all athletes, even the best conditioned and most careful of them. In this chapter, we'll take a look at how good nutrition can speed your recovery and get you back on your feet.

Your Body to the Rescue

If serious enough, injury or illness can put you in the doctor's office. Way before you walk in that door, however, your body has already been doing some doctoring on its own. Your immune system has already snapped to attention and has marshaled its troops to battle whatever it is that is causing you problems.

As you know, your body is composed of a number of systems. Each system plays a different role. The skeletal system, for example, provides support for tissues and muscles, protects vital organs, helps the body move, and stores minerals and immature blood cells. The immune system is the body system that keeps you well.

Foodie

The **immune system** is the body system that protects you against internal damage from pathogens—things like viruses, bacteria, fungi, toxins, and parasites that cause disease and illness when they enter the body. It also helps repair mechanical damage to the body.

Meet Your Immune System

The *immune system* has external and internal components. The skin is the body's primary protection against germs. It is also one of the immune system's most important parts, as well as its largest. The nose, eyes, and mouth also play key roles in germ protection. The substances they contain—tears, mucous, saliva, and mast cells—have factors that break down and kill potential invaders. Any germs trying to enter your body must first make it past all of these defense systems.

Among the millions of germs that you are exposed to on a daily basis, very few are actually able to gain entry into your body. But it can happen, and it does. Sometimes your body lacks the specific defense mechanisms it needs to combat certain germs. Sometimes your immune system isn't strong enough to fight them.

If a germ is successful at getting past this first line of defense, it meets up with more immune system troops inside the body, including the following:

◆ The lymph system, which is a network of vessels, nodes, and organs that drain excess fluid from body tissue and return it to the bloodstream through the heart. Along the way, it detects and removes any bacteria that may have entered the cells. When you go to the doctor because you're not feeling well, one of the first things he or she will check are the lymph nodes in your neck and sometimes in other parts of your body. They aren't usually seen or felt, but if you're battling an infection, these nodes will enlarge, indicating that they're working extra hard to produce white blood cells.

◆ The thymus. This gland is located in your chest between your breastbone and your heart. It produces T-cells, which are another infection fighter. The thymus is an important part of the immune system in newborns, but adults can live without it, as other parts of the immune system can compensate for it.

◆ The spleen. The spleen is another blood filterer. It takes care of foreign cells and old red blood cells that need replacing. People can live without their spleens, but they do so at an increased risk for infection.

◆ Bone marrow. The marrow in your bones is a factory for red and white blood cell production. White blood cells are the ones that battle infection and there are many different kinds of them. The blood cells produced by bone marrow are all based on cells called stem cells, which get their name based on their ability to branch off and turn into many different kinds of cells.

◆ Antibodies. Also called immunoglobulins and gammaglobulins, antibodies are Y-shaped proteins that are produced by white blood cells. Since they are proteins, they differ in how their amino acids are arranged, which means that they also respond differently to different germ cells. Each antibody has special receptors at their tips that are sensitive to specific germs and bind to them in some way. When they bind together, the antibody disables the germ.

◆ The complement system. Complements are blood proteins similar to antibodies that are manufactured in your liver. The complement proteins are so named because antibodies activate them and they work with them. When they find a questionable cell in the body, they burst it open through a process called lysis. This summons white blood cells called phagocytes to the scene, where they clean up the debris from the burst cell as well as any bacteria or other undesirable substances that might be present.

◆ Hormones. Several components of the immune system, such as the thymus gland, generate hormones that play a part in immunity by influencing how other immune cells function.

 Eat It Up! _____

It's important to keep a positive attitude when you're injured or ill. Here's why: When you're afraid, nervous, anxious, angry, or upset, your adrenaline level goes up. As it does, levels of certain hormones called steroids and corticosteroids, which are components of adrenaline, also increase in your body. These hormones suppress the immune system. They can also create a series of metabolic changes that can increase protein loss through the urine. Both can slow down the healing process.

Of the various components of the immune system, white blood cells are probably the most important part. There are many different kinds and they all work together to destroy bacteria and viruses.

When the immune system senses that pathogens have invaded the body, it releases white blood cells from the bone marrow into the bloodstream. The main function of the white blood cells is to surround these body invaders and take them out of the game. White blood cells also:

◆ Detoxify poisons in the body.

◆ Produce and release antibodies and other beneficial chemicals.

◆ Clean up wastes left by other white blood cells.

Foodie

Vasodilation is a widening of the blood vessels, especially the arteries, leading to increased blood flow or reduced blood pressure.

The immune system also comes to the rescue when you're injured. As it does, three things happen:

1. Blood supply to the injured area is increased through a process called *vasodilation*. The injured area will look like it has a larger number of blood vessels. In other words, it will look inflamed and red.

2. The large cells that line the blood vessels retract, which allows more fluids than usual to travel in and out of the capillaries. This both lets larger molecules than usual escape from the capillaries and gives the immune system cells greater access to the injured area. It also lets protein and fluid move into the trauma area. Fibrin is one protein that enters into injured tissue. As it does, it coagulates and becomes trapped. This causes fluid retention—swelling—which inhibits the body's ability to keep the healing process going. In layman's terms, the injured area swells and becomes warm due to increased movement of fluid in and out of the cells.

3. Finally, leukocytes, or white blood cells, move out of the capillaries into the wounded area. In the earliest stages of inflammation, white blood cells called neutrophils, which are responsible for protecting the body against infection, are the most prevalent. Later on, special white blood cells called monocytes and lymphocytes also travel to the infection site. Monocytes are large white blood cells that are formed in the bone marrow and the spleen. They consume large foreign particles and cell debris. Lymphocytes produce antibodies that attack infected cells (cancerous ones, too). The white blood cells break down fibrin and allow the fluid trapped in the area to drain into the lymph system. As this takes place, pressure and pain decrease and eventually go away.

Heating Things Up

Inflammation is your body's first response to physical trauma of any kind. When you sustain an injury, the inflammation is usually pretty obvious—the body part that's injured is painful, warm, and swollen. These are all signs of the white blood cells of the immune system racing to defend and heal the injury. The heat of the inflammation helps the white blood cells do a better job as they work best in a warm environment.

When you're sick, the pathogens that have invaded your body and are now multiplying inside it also cause inflammation. The headaches, muscle aches, fever, chills, and fatigue that you experience when you're ill are caused by the inflammation and the response of the immune system to the pathogens. Another symptom of injury or illness is increased pulse rate, which occurs as the body's metabolism speeds up as part of its infection-fighting mechanism.

The basic goal in managing illness and injury is to give your body's immune system the support it needs to do its job, and to support any repair work that your body has to do on bones and tissue. Part of that support calls for reducing inflammation, as too much of it can retard the healing process. If you've been injured before, you know the routine:

Eat It Up!

Inflammation is swelling, redness, heat, and pain produced in an area of the body as a reaction to injury or infection. The five basic symptoms of inflammation— redness (rubor), swelling (tumour), heat (calor), pain (dolor), and, in severe cases, deranged function (functio laesa) have been known since ancient times.

- Rest. This means taking the injured area out of commission. You have to stop doing whatever caused the injury for a certain period of time.

- Ice. Applying ice, or a cold pack, to an injury for the first 48 to 72 hours will help keep the swelling down. Once the swelling has gone down, you'll want to apply moist heat to the injured area. This helps increase the circulation to the area and speed up repair.

- Compress. Wrapping your injury reduces swelling and keeps the area warm, which will also aid in recovery. You want to wrap the injured area securely, but not so tight as to reduce circulation to the injury.

- Elevate. Elevating your injured part also reduces swelling. Get it up as high as you can, preferably higher than your heart.

Many experts recommend taking an anti-inflammatory medicine, such as ibuprofen, in the first days following an injury. Aspirin, ibuprofen, and acetaminophen are all fever reducers and can also be used for this purpose. However, it's usually a better idea to let a low-grade fever—which indicates that the body is doing its job and fighting whatever has invaded it—run its course. Without fever, the healing process might not get off to a good start or might be less effective than it should be.

> **Dawn Says**
>
> If your body is in optimal nutritional form, you'll have a better foundation for healing damaged muscles, tendons, ligaments, broken bones, or wounds.

Proper nutrition is the other way to support the body when it's ill or injured. While it's always important to eat right, good nutrition is especially important when the body has to heal.

Eating for Healing

Eating when you're injured or sick may be the last thing you feel like doing. Your appetite might be suppressed by pain or medication, or you might simply not be very hungry. However, eating right is the best thing you can do for your body. Good nutrition is vitally important to the healing process. Not only do certain nutrients speed up healing, but you also need to take in enough energy to meet the increased metabolic demands that the healing process places on your body. Depending on the type or severity of the illness or injury, metabolism can speed up to levels that are 20 to 150 percent higher than normal.

> **⚠ CAUTION Food Foul-Ups** _____
>
> When you're under the weather or injured, calorie restriction should be the last thing on your mind unless you're going to be off your feet for a long time. During a severe illness, the body metabolizes everything at a faster rate, and it burns protein faster than it burns fat. The body's need for recovery calories is so strong that a sick person's body may even metabolize and shrink the heart muscle. If you neglect your nutrition, you might tack extra days onto your recovery time.

The basic prescription for eating while you're healing emphasizes the same healthy nutritional balance that comprises normal nutrition. The energy needed for tissue maintenance and repair is supplied by all three macronutrients—carbohydrates, fat, and protein. While protein is vitally important for tissue regeneration, you also need to take in adequate amounts of carbs and fat for energy. Doing so will reserve the protein you eat for the cellular growth that your body needs to heal properly.

As always, choose nutrient-dense foods as much as possible. If you eat animal protein, continue to choose lean meats, such as fish, chicken, and turkey. If you're not hungry, you might find it easier to get your protein by making shakes from protein powder.

> ### Dawn Says
>
> When you're recovering from illness or injury, you might need to increase your protein intake slightly to boost healing. If so, don't increase your portions. Instead, add another serving of protein to your daily menu plan. Spacing out your protein consumption over the course of the day will help your body to better utilize this important macronutrient. If you take in more of it than your body can use at one time, your body might eliminate it instead.

Other tips for eating when recovering from illness or injury include:

◆ Staying away from junk food. Yes, it's comfort food, and it might be just what you need if you're feeling blue. However, taking in empty calories from junk food can keep you from eating the foods that will support your recovery. If you have to indulge, try to minimize the nutritional hit by choosing healthy snacks like frozen fruit bars and low-fat, low-sugar frozen yogurt.

◆ Increasing your fluid intake. Staying hydrated is essential for injury and illness recovery. Dehydration will slow your recovery. Water is the best choice as it doesn't add any calories to your diet. If it doesn't appeal to you, sports drinks are a good alternative. Other options include milk and juice. If possible, try to get your fluids through water or milk. Juice is good, but it tends to be high in simple sugars. Complex carbs are your best choice for this nutrient. Another good hydration booster is soup. Chicken soup, of course, is the classic home remedy for just about any ailment. It's been shown to have measureable health benefits. Not only can it unclog clogged sinuses, it can also reduce inflammation, congestion, and irritation in the airways.

 Eat It Up!

Chicken soup's curative powers have been the focus of studies and scrutiny for some time. According to researchers at the University of Nebraska in Omaha, the wonder soup inhibits certain white blood cells from responding to inflammation, which keeps inflammation levels down and enables the body to heal faster.

◆ Suspending weight-loss efforts (if you're following a calorie-reduced diet). As previously mentioned, recovery from injury or illness often requires more calories to make up for the metabolic changes that are part of the healing process. Trying to lose weight and heal at the same time can slow down the healing process and can also slow your weight loss. While you're recovering, increase the number of calories you take in to a maintenance level.

Taking in adequate levels of all three macronutrients will go a long way toward providing the necessary levels of the micronutrients that are integral to healing and recovery:

◆ Vitamins A, C, and K

◆ The B-complex vitamins, along with folic acid and vitamin B-6

◆ Minerals such as calcium, iron, zinc, copper, manganese, and zinc

Taking a multivitamin/multimineral supplement will ensure that you get enough of these nutrients. Choose one that provides at least 100 percent of the RDA for all minerals, including calcium and magnesium. At the very least, take extra vitamin C, which is important for collagen production as well as antioxidant protection. One way to calculate how much more you should take is by multiplying your body weight by 10; then round this number to the nearest 100. As an example, if you weigh 140, you'll want to take 1,500 mg of vitamin C daily.

Supplementation for Injury Recovery

If you've sustained a significant injury, increasing some nutrients might be necessary due to the increased metabolic stress that your body is going through. Bone injuries, for example, require vitamin K and vitamin D for healing. As previously noted, vitamin C helps make collagen, the protein that reinforces all of the body's connective tissues. If you are concerned about getting enough of these nutrients, it's always wise to give yourself some supplemental insurance.

In recent years, supplements called oral proteolytic enzymes—such as bromelain, which comes from unripe pineapple cores, and papain, which is derived from unripe papaya—have been promoted for treating acute injuries such as bruises, sprains, and strains. These enzymes, which primarily assist protein digestion, are believed to speed healing and diminish inflammation, swelling, and pain by reducing fibrin, which is a protein that the body deposits around an injury to protect the tissue. The idea is to start taking them as soon as possible after an injury is sustained, and to continue taking them throughout the course of recovery and rehabilitation to reduce stress-induced inflammation at the injury site.

The jury is still out on whether these enzymes are all that they're purported to be. Some reports say that proteolytic enzyme therapy has been shown to reduce healing times by up to 50 percent. However, the standard course of treatment in proteolytic enzyme therapy calls for taking these supplements for about three to six weeks, which typically isn't any shorter than the standard recovery time for injuries that aren't serious.

> **Dawn Says**
>
> It's always a good idea to approach any treatment regimen or supplement that promises miraculous recoveries with a healthy dose of skepticism. Proteolytic enzymes might even increase bleeding if they're combined with blood thinners or anti-inflammatory medications like aspirin or ibuprofen, or when taken with vitamin E or gingko biloba. If you're going to try proteolytic enzymes, do so as part of a supervised rehabilitation program.

Dealing with Weight Gain

Athletes always worry about gaining weight when they're off their feet for any length of time. It's a valid concern for some, especially if the recovery period is going to be long. If your injury or illness is going to restrict your activity for less than a week, you won't need to make any drastic changes in your diet, and, in fact, they're not recommended.

If it's going to take you longer than a week to recover, you may need to reduce your food intake to meet your lower energy needs. Be careful, however. Eating too few calories can delay the healing process because your body won't get enough nutrients.

> **Dawn Says**
>
> If you're going to be off your feet for a long time, you might find it helpful to keep a food log to monitor your eating patterns and nutrient intake. While an injury does require time away from the rigors of training and performance, if you're smart about adjusting your nutritional intake during your off time, you'll experience less body-fat increases during the recuperation period. Doing so will let you return to training and competition in close to the same shape you were in before you were benched.

It's important, however, to keep an eye on food intake if you're just a little under the weather. If you're bored and you have time on your hands, you may end up eating more simply because it's there and you don't have anything else to do. If you're feeling anxious about your condition, your feelings can lead to food cravings and to relying on food for comfort. Even if you aren't having special problems with food, you can gain unwanted weight if you continue to follow your usual training diet.

Antioxidants and Injuries

As discussed in Chapter 11, antioxidants are important for protecting the immune system from many damaging stressors, including the effects of intense exercise. They also play an important role in healing. Inflammation can generate large amounts of free radicals, which can damage connective tissue and delay healing. If you're not already taking antioxidant supplements, it can be a very good idea to start doing so as part of your recovery. Look for a product that contains the following antioxidants, which are the ones that are most important for injury recovery:

- Vitamin C
- Vitamin E
- Beta carotene
- Vitamin B-6
- Zinc
- Selenium
- Coenzyme Q10
- Superoxide dismutase and catalase (both are antioxidant enzymes)
- Taurine
- Methionine
- Glutathione
- N-acetylcysteine (also called NAC)

Boosting Your Immune System

The best defense against illness is a good immune system, and one of the best ways to make sure your immunity levels are where they should be is to eat right—to take in the right proportions of nutrients, eat enough of them, and fuel your body with them throughout the day. Supplementation is also key. A good multivitamin/multimineral supplement that emphasizes antioxidants will provide the levels of the micronutrients needed to support your immune system and protect against infection and illness.

A number of nutritional supplements tout their abilities to enhance the immune system and fight infection. While it's always a good idea to take such claims with a grain of salt, it's also important to realize that we still don't know a great deal about what many of these substances can do. However, thanks to ongoing nutritional research, we're learning more about them all the time. Still, you're going to see conflicting information about many of them, which can make it difficult to determine what works and what doesn't. Glutamine, for example, is one product that is often spotlighted as aiding faster recovery and boosting immune function. It is true that glutamine levels drop during exercise, but it would take massive amounts of intense activity to deplete the body's glutamine stores enough to diminish immune function. For this reason, many experts believe that glutamine supplementation isn't necessary. However, there is research that supports its benefits for all-around cellular support and recovery from exercise.

How can you know what to use? Consulting with a sports nutritionist is always a good idea when you're looking for ways to boost your performance, prevent injuries, or heal from them after they happen. Doing your own research is always better than relying on advertising claims. You'll find some resources to help you in Appendix B.

The simplest and best way to protect against illness is to be wise about your training and eating practices. If you train too hard before competition, you might weaken your immune system and open yourself up for illness. Not eating right can have the same effects on your body.

Eating carbohydrates during intense and lengthy exercise—lasting longer than 90 minutes—is a proven nutritional practice that will enhance immune function. Here's why: Carbohydrates, as you know, metabolize into glucose, and glucose is what fuels immune cells. When you keep glucose levels high, immune levels stay high with them. When blood glucose levels drop, the immune cells don't get the fuel they need to function properly. Low blood glucose levels also trigger the release of stress hormones, which further suppress immune function.

> **Eat It Up!** _____
>
> Endurance athletes aren't more susceptible to getting colds or flu than the average, more sedentary person. But there may be a window of time of approximately 3 to 72 hours after an intense workout or race that the immune system is weakened. This gives viruses and bacteria a greater opportunity to attack.

> **Dawn Says**
>
> If you are prone to injuries or illness, take a look at your sleeping habits. It's hard to train a tired body, which is what you have when you don't get enough sleep. Athletes compensate well for lack of sleep because their bodies are in better shape, but consistently pushing yourself beyond your limits can bring on illness and cause injury. If you don't get enough sleep on a regular basis, try to eliminate sleep wasters from your schedule. And take naps!

If you let your blood sugar drop too low during long, intense workouts or competitions—marathons or triathalons are good examples of these—you also reduce your resistance to viruses and bacteria. This period of low resistance can last anywhere from 3 to 72 hours, which is plenty of time for germs to gang up on you and gain entry into your body.

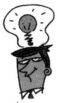

Eat It Up! _____

Runners who quaff sports drinks during long periods of hard exercise have been shown to be more resistant to exercise-related illnesses than those who drink plain water.

Eat It Up! _____

Studies show that regular exercise can decrease upper respiratory tract infections. Researchers compared the health records of two groups of women. One group exercised five days a week for 45 minutes each session. The other didn't. The number of upper respiratory tract infections was significantly less in the group that exercised.

The best way to keep from getting ill during these periods is to keep your blood sugar levels up to where they should be when you're competing. This means regularly taking in carbohydrates to replenish your glycogen supplies.

Exercise itself is a powerful immune system builder. Not only are immune levels higher in people who exercise on a regular basis, but exercise has also been shown to boost the level of natural killer (NK) and T helper cells in the body that suppress certain types of cancer. What better testimony is there to the benefits of staying in good shape?

However, while some exercise is good, too much exercise can have a negative effect. Overtraining is a serious problem for many athletes, as it can wear the body down, especially if recovery times between workouts aren't sufficient. It can also double the risk of getting sick. When too much exercise is combined with insufficient recovery times, not enough sleep, too much stress, and not eating the right foods or not eating enough of them, the chances of getting sick or injured substantially increase. In exercise as well as nutrition, balance is key. Combining both in healthy amounts is an unbeatable prescription for preventing disease and living a long, healthy life.

The Least You Need to Know

- Recovering from illness or injury requires eating a well-balanced diet of nutrient-rich foods.

- Long recoveries may require adjusting calorie intake to compensate for reduced physical activity.

- There are no "magic potions" that will speed up recovery. Take any claims of products that can do so with a grain of salt.

- The best way to boost your immunity is to exercise regularly and eat a balanced diet.

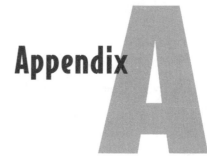

Appendix A

Glossary

amenorrhea   The absence or surpression of menstruation.

anemia   The blood condition in which there are too few red blood cells, or the red blood cells are deficient in hemoglobin.

atrophic gastritis   The inability to produce stomach acid.

basal metabolic rate (BMR)   The amount of energy your body needs to fuel itself while at complete rest.

body mass index (BMI)   A formula that uses weight and height to estimate body fat.

calorie   The measure of the energy contained in food. One calorie is the amount of energy it takes to increase the temperature of 1 gram of water 1 degree Centigrade.

dietary supplements   Products that contain a vitamin, a mineral, an herb or other botanical, an amino acid, or a dietary substance used to supplement the diet by increasing total daily intake.

electrolytes   Electrically charged particles, or ions, that regulate fluid exchange in the body's cells and blood.

extracellular fluids   Fluids found outside of the cells of the body. Also called interstitial fluids.

fat-soluble vitamins   Vitamins that dissolve in fat.

female athlete triad The combination of athletic amenorrhea, disordered eating, and premature osteoporosis.

heme iron The type of iron found in animal protein.

immune system The bodily system that protects you against internal damage from pathogens—things like viruses, bacteria, fungi, and parasites that cause disease and illness when they enter the body. It also helps repair mechanical damage to the body.

intracellular fluids Fluids that are found inside the cells of the body.

macrominerals The seven minerals that the body needs large amounts of.

metabolism The process of chemical digestion and its related reactions that provide the energy and nutrients needed to sustain life.

microminerals Minerals that the body needs in smaller amounts.

microtrace minerals Minerals that the body needs in very small amounts.

nonheme iron Iron that comes from sources other than animal protein.

nutrients Nourishing substances that are essential to life.

nutrition A science that deals with foods and their effect on health.

physiology The branch of biology that deals with the internal workings of living things, including such functions as metabolism, respiration, and reproduction.

protein Comes from the Greek word "proteios," meaning "of prime importance."

sports nutrition A science that deals with food and how it affects the health and performance of athletes.

vasodilation A widening of the blood vessels, and especially the arteries, leading to increased blood flow or reduced blood pressure.

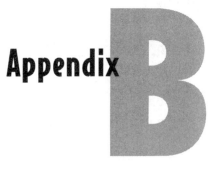

Appendix B

Resources

On the Web

Coupons

The following sites offer coupons for food and other products.

www.coolsavings.com

www.funnytummy.com

www.blueballweb.net/Groceries.html

www.momsview.com/foodcoupons.html

www.valpak.com

www.couponclearinghouse.com

www.theentertainmentcouponbook.com

www.valupage.com

www.200freebies.com

www.memolink.com

Nutrition Information

Check out these sites for more information on a variety of subjects related to food and nutrition.

www.nal.usda.gov/fnic/cgi-bin/nut_search.pl

This is a searchable nutrient database sponsored by the USDA's Agricultural Research Service.

www.arborcom.com

Founded in 1996 by Australian physician and nutritionist Tony Helman. Provides an annotated listing of links to nearly 3,000 Internet resources covering food, food science, and applied and clinical nutrition.

www.supplementinfo.org

The website for the Dietary Supplement Information Bureau, the online information service of the Dietary Supplement Education Alliance. Good information on this industry, including regulations, and links to more information on dietary supplements.

www.supplementwatch.com

Website full of info on supplements.

www.glycemicindex.com

Searchable GI database, information on GI, research, books, testing services, and more.

www.50plus.org

The website for the Fifty-Plus organization, dedicated to the health and fitness needs of seniors who exercise to stay in shape.

www.soyfoods.com

Want to learn more about soy? This website is packed with information on the different types of soy foods and has a good list of recipes for cooking with soy.

www.usana.com

Complete vitamin, mineral, and antioxidant formulas for all adults, teenagers, and children. Advanced dosages promote long-term health; highest quality ingredients selected for potency, purity, and bioavailablity, documented safety, designed for convenience, compliance, and results. Designed and manufactured according to

USP and pharmaceutical GMP guidelines. Contact Clairinda 513-521-4376 or toll-free at 1-877-202-1026 or email www.unitoday.net/clairinda

www.sportsnutritiontogo.com

Maximizes sports nutrition goals for all types of athletes, recreational to professional. Sports Nutrition to Go! works with each individual to maintain ideal body composition, maximize concentration, minimize fatigue, reduce errors, decrease injuries, maximize recovery, decrease the use of harmful supplements and illegal substances, and increase longevity in the sport. Contact Dawn at 513-521-4376 or e-mail sportsnutritiontogo@hotmail.com

www.muscleactivation.com

A dynamic approach to treating muscular imbalances that will reduce or eliminate pain and fatigue and speed muscle recovery. A noninvasive methodology for improving everyday activities for all age groups and body types. Allows the body to achieve optimal functionality, without pain or injury, by increasing the body's range of motion, restoring muscular alignment, and eliminating compensation patterns. A checks and balances system designed to identify and treat the causes of chronic pain and injury. Contact Sheila Lee at 859-866-0739 or e-mail denaligirl@fuse.net

www.aweighout.com

Classes, groups, and individual coaching services for people who want to learn new strategies to combat emotional eating (eating when stressed, anxious, bored, angry, etc.). Services provided both in-person in the Cincinnati area and by telephone nationwide. Contact info@aweighout.com or call 513-321-7202.

Print Resources

The following books and magazines cover a wide range of nutrition and sports nutrition topics.

Cameron, Julia. *The Artist's Way*. New York: Jeremy P. Tarcher/Putnam, 1992.

Books

Balch, James F. and Balch, Phyllis A. *Prescription for Nutritional Healing: A Practical A-Z Reference to Drug-Free Remedies Using Vitamins, Minerals, Herbs, and Food Supplements, 3rd Edition*. New York: Avery Penguin Putnam, 2000.

Bean, Anita. *Food for Fitness: Nutrition Guide, Eating Plans, over 200 Recipes.* London: A&C Black, 1998.

Clark, Nancy. *Nancy Clark's Sports Nutrition Guidebook, 2nd Edition.* Champaign, Illinois: Human Kinetics, 1996.

Coleman, Ellen, and Steen, Suzanne Nelson. *Ultimate Sports Nutrition Handbook, 2nd Edition.* Palo Alto, Calif.: Bull Pub. Co., 2000.

Evans, William, and Rosenberg, Irwin H. Biomarkers: *The 10 Keys to Prolonging Vitality.* New York: Fireside Publishing, 1992.

Kleiner, Susan M. *Power Eating, 2nd Edition.* Champaign, Illinois: Human Kinetics, 2001.

MacWilliam, Lyle. *The Comparative Guide to Nutritional Supplements, 3rd Edition.* Vernon, B.C.: Northern Dimensions Publishing.

Peterson, Marilyn. *Eat to Compete, 2nd Edition.* St. Louis: Mosby, 1996.

Strand, Ray D. *What Your Doctor Doesn't Know About Nutritional Medicine May Be Killing You.* Nashville, Tenn.: Thomas Nelson, 2003.

Weatherwax, Dawn. *The Official Snack Guide for Beleaguered Sports Parents.* Cincinnati, Ohio: WellCentered Books, 2001.

Williams, Melvin H. *The Ergogenics Edge.* Champaign, Ill.: Human Kinetics, 1998.

Wood, Christine. *How to Get Kids to Eat Great & Love It!, 2nd Edition.* Irvine, Calif.: Griffin Publishing, 2001.

Magazines and Newsletters

Cooking Light
www.cookinglight.com

Nutrition Action Healthletter
www.cspinet.org/nah/

Vegetarian Times
www.vegetariantimes.com

Associations

The following associations provide information on various aspects of health, nutrition, and keeping fit.

American Cancer Society
1-800-227-2345
www.cancer.org/help.html

American Sport Education Program
1-800-747-5698

The American Diabetes Association
703-549-1500
www.oso.com/community/groups/diabetes/index.html

The American Dietetic Association
1-800-877-1600
www.eatright.org

The American Heart Association
1-800-242-8721
www.americanheart.org

Gatorade Sports Institute
1-800-616-4774
www.gssiweb.com

National Strength and Conditioning Association
1-888-746-2378
www.nsca-cc.org

National Athletic Trainers' Association
1-800-711-7928
www.nata.org

Index

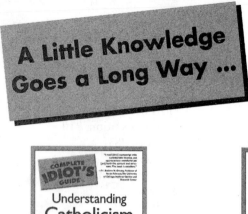
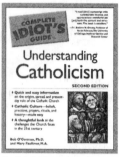
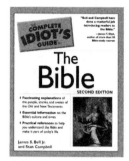
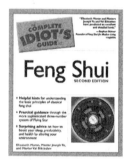
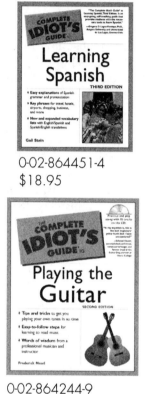
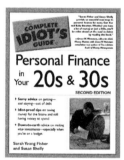
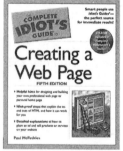
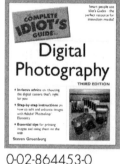
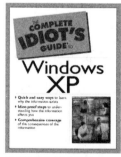